Acclaim for
Are You Coming?

"Sex-positive, empowering, and easy to read. If you want to learn more about how to harness your body's capacity for pleasure and orgasm, read this book!"
—**Dr. Laurie Mintz,** author of *Becoming Cliterate: Why Orgasm Equality Matters—And How to Get It*

"Why the long wait for this book? *Are You Coming?* ought to be on every woman's reading list. I bet that more than half of this book will come as a surprise to them. And let's be honest, men ought to read this too. It's easy enough because the writing is really accessible (and the gorgeous illustrations are a great help too)."—**VIVA Magazine**

"Manages to make sense of the most surprising sexual topics— and in a highly creative way. . . . Entertaining and useful!" —**Amayzine**

Are You
Coming?

Are You Coming?

A Vagina Owner's Guide to Orgasm

Laura Hiddinga

Illustrations by Bo Sterenberg

THE EXPERIMENT

NEW YORK

ARE YOU COMING?: *A Vagina Owner's Guide to Orgasm*
Copyright © 2019, 2021 by LotteLust/Laura Hiddinga/Kosmos Uitgevers
Illustrations copyright © 2019, 2021 by Bo Sterenberg
Translation, as well as text on pp. 76–81, copyright © 2021 by The Experiment, LLC

Originally published in the Netherlands as *Kom je ook?* by Kosmos Uitgevers, Utrecht/Antwerp, an imprint of VBK | media, in 2019. First published in English in North America in revised form by The Experiment, LLC, in 2020.

The Experiment, LLC
220 East 23rd Street, Suite 600
New York, NY 10010-4658
theexperimentpublishing.com

This book contains the opinions and ideas of its author. It is intended to provide helpful and informative material on the subjects addressed in the book. It is sold with the understanding that the author and publisher are not engaged in rendering medical, health, or any other kind of personal professional services in the book. The author and publisher specifically disclaim all responsibility for any liability, loss, or risk—personal or otherwise—that is incurred as a consequence, directly or indirectly, of the use and application of any of the contents of this book.

THE EXPERIMENT and its colophon are registered trademarks of The Experiment, LLC. Many of the designations used by manufacturers and sellers to distinguish their products are claimed as trademarks. Where those designations appear in this book and The Experiment was aware of a trademark claim, the designations have been capitalized.

The Experiment's books are available at special discounts when purchased in bulk for premiums and sales promotions as well as for fund-raising or educational use. For details, contact us at info@theexperimentpublishing.com.

Library of Congress Cataloging-in-Publication Data
Names: Hiddinga, Laura, author. | Sterenberg, Bo, 1998- illustrator.
Title: Are you coming? : a vagina owner's guide to orgasm / Laura Hiddinga
  ; illustrations by Bo Sterenberg.
Other titles: Kom je ook? English
Description: New York, NY : The Experiment, LLC, 2020. | "Originally
  published in the Netherlands as Kom je ook? by Kosmos Uitgevers,
  Utrecht/Antwerp, an imprint of VBK | media, in 2019"--Title page verso.
Identifiers: LCCN 2020035584 (print) | LCCN 2020035585 (ebook) | ISBN
  9781615197088 | ISBN 9781615197095 (ebook)
Subjects: LCSH: Sex instruction for women. | Female orgasm.
Classification: LCC HQ46 .H49 2020 (print) | LCC HQ46 (ebook) | DDC
  613.9/6082--dc23
LC record available at https://lccn.loc.gov/2020035584
LC ebook record available at https://lccn.loc.gov/2020035585

ISBN 978-1-61519-708-8
Ebook ISBN 978-1-61519-709-5

Cover and text design by Beth Bugler
Author photograph by Nikki Okker
Translated by Laura Vroomen

Manufactured in Turkey

First printing February 2021
10 9 8 7 6 5 4 3 2 1

Contents

Introduction

I*t's a crying shame. Between the sheets, heterosexual women are consistently shortchanged. And that's no exaggeration! According to a 2016 report published in the *Archives of Sexual Behavior*, only 65 percent of straight women climax during sex, while 95 percent of their male partners always enjoy a happy ending. (But in other studies, the figure for straight women has been as low as 35 percent!) Compare this to the 86 percent of lesbian women who reported "nearly always" or "always" experiencing orgasm. And for people who've undergone gender confirmation surgery, it's an issue, too: In one study of male-to-female patients post-operation, around 19 percent reported they "rarely easily" achieve orgasm during sex. Nearly 43 percent said they "usually easily" achieve orgasm—but "usually" is hard to define. And it definitely doesn't mean *always*!

Why this orgasm chasm? Judging by quite a few studies, many men believe that women can come through penetration alone. In reality, only about a quarter have that gift. But we also need to take a long hard look at ourselves, because some of us vagina owners tend to put our own pleasure second—and no matter what our sexual orientation is. We're not familiar enough with our pleasure spots, don't issue instructions, and, for many straight women especially, settle for a short bout of "foreplay." (See the sidebar "What counts as sex?" on page 14 if you want to know why I put this term in quotation marks!)

This book is going to change that—or rather, you are. In the next 200 pages, you'll be learning *everything* you need to know when it comes to the basic guidelines for orgasm. How does an orgasm really work? What types of orgasms are there and how do you get them? How do you deal with pain during sex? Why do you get there so much faster solo than with someone else? How do you give your bed partner(s) feedback? In short: How does your sex life get better, hotter, more fun?

And feel free to leave this book lying around in the bedroom for your sex partner to stumble across. Who knows, they may learn a thing or two!

A note before you get started

We have done our best to use inclusive language in this book, but unfortunately widely reported research on sex is not as inclusive as it could be: The focus has predominately been on "women" and "men" without consideration of alternative gender identities and often in heterosexual relationships. Even less consider trans people's experiences. While we use inclusive language as much as possible, in order to accurately reference source material, we have maintained the terminology used ("women," "men") in historical and scientific research.

The terms "assigned female at birth" (AFAB) and "assigned male at birth" (AMAB) also appear throughout. For those unfamiliar: Because some people do not identify with the gender assigned to them at birth and are gender nonconforming and/or transgender or gender-expansive, this is the preferred term to refer to someone who was born with "female" or "male" genitals.

And to our readers recovering from surgery of any kind, please remember: Your body needs to recover fully before you experiment with any techniques in this book! If in doubt, consult with your doctor.

1

Orgasm:
the basics

*What they don't teach you
in history and biology class*

"What's the big mystery? It's my clitoris, not the Sphinx."

Miranda Hobbes in
Sex and the City

In search of the clitoris

When it comes to orgasm, the clitoris is the star—the ancient Greeks and Romans already knew that. And yet, for centuries the holy clit has been marginalized. It was found, then cast aside, before being discovered all over again.

The quest for the divine Big O goes back at least as far as the Stone Age when homemade stone (!) sex toys were made. Cleopatra (69 BCE–30 BCE) is said to have inserted gourds filled with bees into her vagina, and Marie Bonaparte (1882–1962) had her clitoris surgically repositioned no fewer than three times so she'd climax more easily during sex. Whether either of these was a success or not, it certainly shows that curiosity about the "mysterious female orgasm" has been a hot topic since time immemorial.

That makes it all the more bizarre that the clitoris's function wasn't discovered until 1998. One of the men to blame for this is Sigmund Freud. The neurologist was familiar with the pleasure bud, but in 1905 he reckoned that "we" don't need to pay it all that much attention. Clitoral orgasms were the reserve of inexperienced adolescent girls. A real, mature woman came through vaginal stimulation, or so he concluded. Boy, was he wrong!

This is why masturbation was long considered to be totally unacceptable. People thought it could make you mentally and physically ill—and even lead to premature death. Yet vagina owners knew better. A study published in 1953 found that 62 percent

"The study of sex is the beginning of all life. Yet we sit like prudish cavemen in the dark riddled with shame and guilt"

Dr. William Masters in the TV series *Masters of Sex*

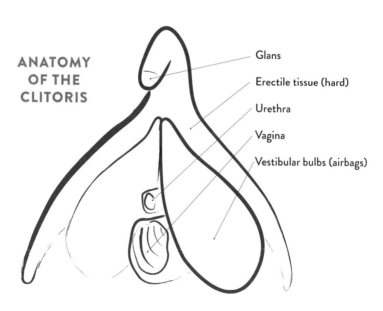

ANATOMY OF THE CLITORIS

Glans

Erectile tissue (hard)

Urethra

Vagina

Vestibular bulbs (airbags)

of women touched themselves; in 1979 the figure rose to 74 percent. The myth was finally debunked in 1988 by the legendary sex researchers William Masters and Virginia Johnson, who built off of Alfred Kinsey's research. They delivered the liberating news that the clitoris, *not* the vagina, is the big star of our orgasms.

Since ancient Roman times, scientists have been saying every couple of centuries that the clitoris is more than just the outer tip. But for lack of modern medical equipment, this never went beyond mere theorizing. The clitoris was "officially" discovered in 1559 by the Italian Matteo Realdo Colombo. After thousands of dissections he managed to map the internal part of the clitoris—invisible to the naked eye. In 1844, another detailed drawing of

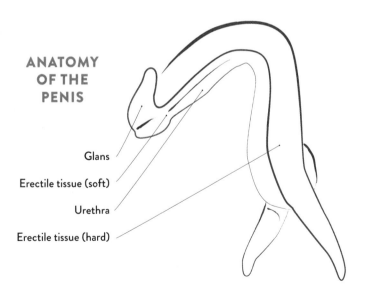

ANATOMY OF THE PENIS

Glans

Erectile tissue (soft)

Urethra

Erectile tissue (hard)

the internal and external clitoris appeared, this one done by George Ludwig Kobelt, a German anatomist. But again and again, the evidence was buried in the medical literature. We're looking at you, Freud.

The year 1998 marks the moment when the true nature of the "tickler" was finally acknowledged and embraced. With the help of new technology (an MRI scan), Australian urologist Helen O'Connell discovered that the pleasure organ is actually a further four inches bigger than previously thought. What you see on the outside is just the tip of the iceberg. The clitoris extends deep inside the body, containing erectile tissue that swells on excitement and surrounds the vagina. Overall, the anatomy of the clitoris looks a lot like that of the penis. That's no surprise, since every penis begins life as a clitoris. When, twelve weeks into a pregnancy, hormones determine that the fetus will become a penis owner, the clitoris develops into a phallus. So although the clitoris predates the penis, the intimate little bud continues to fight for recognition and above all . . . attention.

The difference between the vagina and the vulva

When you say "vagina," do you mean the whole package? I.e., the inner and outer labia, the clitoris, and the urethral orifice? In popular parlance, we tend to use the words vagina and vulva interchangeably. But they're not synonymous. The difference between the two is really quite simple. Here it is: The vagina is the internal part of our sex organ; the vulva is the external part. The vagina consists of the elastic canal between the opening of the vagina and the cervix. The vulva is made up of the labia, glands, clitoris, and the openings of the urethra and the vagina. In other words, everything you can see on the outside.

An orgasm on prescription

It's strange, but true. We owe the invention of the vibrator to ignorant men and "crazy" women. It all began in the thirteenth century, when women sought medical help for that age-old phenomenon known as "hysteria"—an umbrella term for a whole array of mental "problems" like depression, anger, and sexual excess.

Doctors were at their wits' end: Not a single medication worked. Until they discovered, in 1653, that massaging the clitoris offered a solution. It gave these "hysterics" a so-called *paroxysm,* better known as the *orgasm.* But masturbation was strictly forbidden in those days. Making a woman climax was the reserve of husbands and . . . doctors. You get it: Vagina owners were lining up for the hands-on treatment. It should come as no surprise that the doctors got cramps in their fingers as they performed the time-consuming job. They had to do something. And this is how the precursor to the vibrator came about.

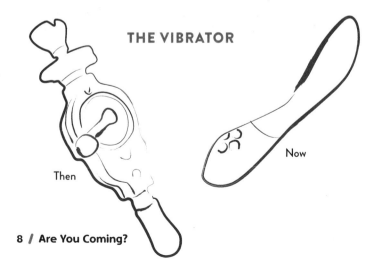

THE VIBRATOR

Then

Now

The so-called massager was hand-operated; later, in the nineteenth century, it was steam driven for hands-free joy. The gadget came to be marketed as a beauty must-have, with the vibrations said to work wonders for wrinkles, neck pain, and circulation. Yeah right. In the early days it looked more like a torture device than a pleasure-giver, but over time it came to resemble the dildos as we now know them: phallic, flexible, and available in all colors of the rainbow.

> ## Quickie
> **Some people have a larger clitoris than others. This has no positive or negative impact on the climax or its intensity, except that the little bud may be a bit easier to locate.**

The uses of an orgasm

It should be clear by now: The female orgasm was suppressed for centuries, in part because of the mystery surrounding the clitoris and in part because there didn't seem to be a reason for it. A happy ending wasn't thought to be necessary for women. For a long time, sex for pleasure wasn't a given. It was a way to make babies. From this evolutionary standpoint, it made sense. Put bluntly: The whole point of a male orgasm was to fire sperm cells at a woman's egg. A woman didn't need a climax for fertilization to happen . . . right?

Not quite. First of all, some scientists believe that way back when (think more than 75 million years ago) a woman needed to orgasm during sex in order to trigger the release of an egg. But in 1850, ovulation was discovered—that's to say, the spontaneous egg release unprompted by external factors. So a woman coming was not, or no longer, essential for procreation.

Well, think again. . . . An orgasm does have a role to play if you're a vagina owner who's trying to get pregnant. You can boost your chances of fertilization by coming either simultaneously or shortly after your partner. Your vagina's contractions help give the sperm cells a push in the right direction (the uterus). But why the clitoris glans is located outside the vaginal entrance remains a mystery. Perhaps it's for the best, because what if the visible clitoris was inside the vagina? Imagine how much more painful childbirth would be if a baby's head scraped past 8,000 additional nerve endings?

Other benefits of orgasm

It goes without saying that another reason for coming is the pleasure it gives. Your *petite mort* releases the feel-good hormones dopamine and oxytocin into your body. These bring you closer to your bed partner and make you feel happy. A climax also boosts your immune system and lowers the risk of cancer and heart disease. It increases blood flow to the brain, so it receives more oxygen and minerals; enhances fertility and stabilizes the menstrual cycle; and increases sex drive, too: Regular orgasms teach your brain that sex is a reward. And did I mention that it also reduces stress, can act as pain relief, and to top it all off, can basically be as effective as a sleeping pill? Orgasms are a wonderful thing.

How does an orgasm work?

To better understand your body, it's good to know how it all works. For example, which visible and invisible changes happen in your body during sex? An orgasm doesn't just appear out of nowhere. To start with, you need to be "in the mood." According to sexologists William Masters and Virginia Johnson, there are four stages of sexual arousal: excitement, plateau, orgasm, and resolution. Other sex researchers, among them Helen Singer Kaplan, later added the phase of "desire."

Desire
Sex and/or an orgasm begins with a desire. An unconscious or conscious stimulus gives you butterflies. What gets you going is different for everybody. For some, it only takes a sensual touch, while others need more stimuli. These may include: a (sexual) fantasy, an exciting DM, an erotic story, a sexy (porn) film, giving or receiving a massage, kissing . . . you name it.

Excitement
In this phase you spring into action: This includes "foreplay," but also full-on sex. Your body will be telling you. Maybe you get wet, you start to feel warm(er), your nipples go hard, you breathe faster, or your heart is pounding.

The other thing that happens, but you're probably unaware of: For those assigned female at birth (AFAB), the breasts grow bigger (up to 25 percent), tissues in the clitoris swell, the vagina widens a little, the cervix is pulled up and out of the way, and the inner labia turn a darker color and become engorged. The skin can go red in places, too: the so-called sex flush.

AFAB or not, it's good to know that the symptoms associated with excitement differ from person to person. While one self-lubricates very easily, another may get really wet just before or after their (first) orgasm . . . even though they're both equally turned on. On average, it takes around twenty minutes before you're aroused enough to be physically ready for penetration and/or working toward a climax. That's why it's so important to take the time for mental and physical arousal.

Jamie: Why don't they ever make a movie about what happens after they kiss? Dylan: They do. It's called porn.

Jamie and Dylan in
Friends with Benefits

What counts as sex?

The dictionary definition of sex is "sexual intercourse": a broad term if ever there was one. But in real life, the word is often synonymous with penetration or coitus: penis inside vagina. Very confusing—not to mention wrong—since this description often excludes queer partners. What's often described, by the media for instance, as "foreplay" for straight partners (like kissing and manual and oral sex) can be appetizer, entrée, and dessert in one for queer ones. Besides, the definition of sex as penetration contributes to the idea that female pleasure is an afterthought and that the male orgasm is what it's all about, since only a handful of people can climax through penetration alone. The conclusion: Manual and oral are sex, too!

When the erectile tissue in the clitoris becomes fully engorged, it's known as an erection. Yup, that's right, you can get a "hard-on," too.

Plateau

During the "plateau phase" all the physical symptoms of the previous excitement stage mount in intensity. Your vagina and clitoris become more sensitive, your heart is pounding even harder, and you're breathing faster and faster.

Orgasm

And then we get to what it's (often, though not always!) all about: the great deliverance. With the right stimulation of the clitoris, vagina, G-spot, breasts, and maybe the cervix, we build up to maximum sexual arousal and from there to a climax and release. In one fell swoop you feel like the happiest person alive thanks to the hit of happy hormones dopamine and oxytocin. All the tension that's been building is released. Muscles around the body rhythmically contract. These contractions are especially intense inside the vagina, cervix, and anus, but some people find that their whole bodies are literally convulsing. And unlike most AMAB penis owners, vagina owners are capable of adding another climax: multiple orgasm. A penis needs to recover before starting all over again at phase one. That clearly gives us the edge. You've never managed this? No worries. You can read more about it in chapter 2.

Resolution

After all this physical exertion and subsequent release, you need time to recover. Your breathing slowly goes back to normal, your muscles relax, your vagina and cervix (if you have one) revert to their original state, and eventually your flushed cheeks fade. Whoever fancies another round can start from scratch again.

> ### Quickie
> **You can also have wet dreams that culminate in an orgasm: In one study, 37 percent of women said this had happened to them.**

Keep it clean!

Whether you're doing it with a partner or solo, it's important that you "keep it clean": Wash your hands before you have sex, use condoms, never go from anal to vaginal penetration (more about this on page 39), and pee after sex—but *not* before!—to flush everything out and prevent bacteria from infecting your urethra. The same goes for your partners—whether it's a person or a toy, make sure they stay clean, too. Toys should be cleaned with a toy cleaner before and after use, as well as when switching between partners if you're having sex with multiple people. And remember: You and your bed partner(s) should be getting tested for STDs on a regular basis.

2

The thirteen types of orgasm

Collect them all!

"To me, sex is power. It's empowering when you do it because you want to do it."

Rihanna in *ELLE* magazine

*T*here isn't just one way to come. There are lots of different ways—no fewer than *thirteen* types of orgasm. Some are like an eruption, others more like a wave. If this sounds like a lot of hard work, remember: There are no obligations. Sex is fun, and we're going to keep it that way.

The basics

Whatever orgasm you're aiming for, some basic conditions need to be met before you can reach any kind of climax.

Desire

Have you ever jumped in the sack when you weren't really in the mood? Then you must have noticed that everything was just that little bit less enjoyable. Without desire you can't get excited, and without physical and mental excitement, an orgasm is unlikely.

Sometimes you'll feel desire in response to unconscious stimuli. Without fully realizing it, the sight of a raunchy film scene, a beautiful chest, or the muscular biceps of a passerby will get things throbbing between your legs. Often it's not that "spontaneous." You don't feel the urge to rip someone's clothes off at a snap of the fingers. You need stimulation.

Excitement builds with the help of visual and/or physical stimuli. What turns you on is personal to you. While some might respond to a porn clip, others get all fired up by an erotic story or their own vivid imagination.

One thing is for sure: the greater the desire, the greater the sexual arousal of body and mind, the greater the chance of an orgasm. That's why maximum arousal is so important. Even when you're going solo, you can have "foreplay" to achieve this. Maybe caress your thighs or massage your breasts or nipples. Discover what turns you on and share it with a partner at a later stage.

Relaxation

A tumble in the sack is an ideal de-stresser, but sometimes stress prevents you from enjoying yourself in bed. Worries about work, personal issues, or other circumstances stop you from focusing on what's happening inside your body. You feel uncomfortable and you can't fully relax. The result? You can't get excited and wet enough, so sex may hurt and you may not be able to reach a climax.

So "switch off" your head before you get intimate! That's obviously easier said than done. But you can start by tidying up the room and taking a warm shower or a hot bath. Create a nice atmosphere. A sultry tune (The Weeknd, Sade, or Marvin Gaye always hits the spot for me), scented candles, and a massage can also be effective. Whatever floats your boat.

You can also create an "ambiance" for yourself when you're masturbating. In fact, it's especially important to set aside plenty of time when you're exploring your own sexuality. "Me time," as it's called. Self-love starts with taking good care of yourself. Indulge in a nice long shower or bath, lather up with your favorite shower gel, and gently scrub your skin. Whether you slip on a racy playsuit or PJs, that's entirely up to you. Choose something that makes you feel good.

Underlying emotions can also get in the way of an orgasm and pleasurable sex. These include bad experiences and taboos surrounding sex, problems in the relationship, lack of self-confidence, etc. We'll look at this in more detail in chapter 6.

Mindset

Your mindset is a powerful tool during sex—if it's used to positive effect. Daunting? Sure. But it's not mission impossible. Try thinking: I've never done this before, but I *know* I can do it. Be your own best friend and have faith in yourself—and, if applicable, in the other person. Push all other conflicting thoughts away, focus on yourself and on your body, and think only of what you find sexy. You deserve it!

Take your time

The general consensus is that it takes us vagina owners an average of twenty minutes to reach orgasm. It's often a bit faster while flying solo. Does it take much longer or shorter for you? Twenty minutes is the average, so there will always be outliers of five minutes or an hour. The length of time differs per person and per occasion. So don't be hurried along by your bed partner. Your orgasm isn't something to be ticked off or rushed through. It's really all about enjoying it to the max. It's important to give good instructions, whether it's a one-night stand, a new flame, or a long-term relationship. We'll come back to this in chapter 4.

Keep practicing

If you're not quite getting there, don't be discouraged. Be realistic. Putting too much pressure on yourself will only be counterproductive. You'll get frustrated with yourself and maybe with your bed partner. You might become negative, impatient, and tense. Sex can be satisfying without an orgasm, too. When all you do is focus on the destination, you forget to enjoy the beautiful views along the way.

"Do you guys know they want me to do a story on a 45-minute orgasm? As if. I mean, by definition they're short and intense, right? For me, they are."

Alice Pieszecki in *The L Word*

Is there such a thing as the libido?

The libido is often described as a primal urge. That's incorrect. A sex drive isn't of the same order as an appetite. Testosterone doesn't actually generate desire by itself. That's all down to the person, not to their sex. But your brain and genitals do need the hormone to respond to sexual stimuli. That's why the idea that men are more interested in sex because they have more testosterone is incorrect. That said, their feedback from genitals to brain is faster, so they're generally quicker to acknowledge their sexual desires. They see their erection and think, "Hey, I want to have sex." For many vagina owners there will be times when their body is aroused (the clitoris is engorged), yet their brain doesn't realize it. According to research by psychologist and sex expert Emily Nagowski, "spontaneous desire" is the reason for sex in only 10 to 20 percent of women compared to around 70 percent of men.

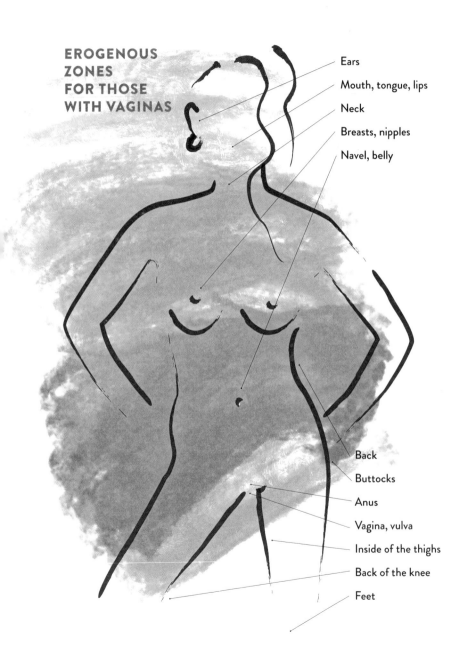

EROGENOUS ZONES FOR THOSE WITH VAGINAS

Ears

Mouth, tongue, lips

Neck

Breasts, nipples

Navel, belly

Back

Buttocks

Anus

Vagina, vulva

Inside of the thighs

Back of the knee

Feet

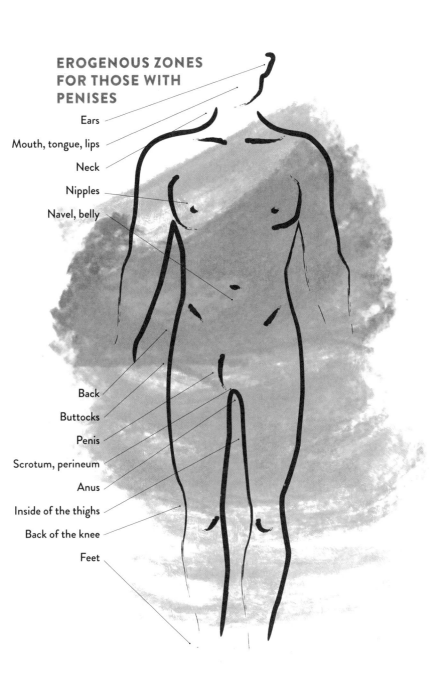

EROGENOUS ZONES FOR THOSE WITH PENISES

Ears

Mouth, tongue, lips

Neck

Nipples

Navel, belly

Back

Buttocks

Penis

Scrotum, perineum

Anus

Inside of the thighs

Back of the knee

Feet

"Only men have vaginal orgasms"

According to the research, only 10 to 20 percent of women come through penetration alone. It's what we call a vaginal orgasm. But that term is incorrect. According to Dutch sexologist Ellen Laan, only straight men have vaginal orgasms . . . when they come inside a vagina. Are you still with me? Here's how it works. As you read in chapter 1, the clitoris is bigger than you can see with the naked eye. The pleasure organ branches out into erectile tissue that surrounds the vagina. When you're aroused, this becomes engorged so the clitoris may be stimulated from inside the vagina, and in some cases even via the anus. The size and position of these branches vary from person to person. The closer they are to the neighboring vagina, the greater the chance that you can come via penetration alone. We call it a vaginal orgasm, but in reality it's the clitoris that's being stimulated. For lack of a better term—and to keep things simple—we refer to it as a vaginal orgasm in this book.

Clitoral orgasm

❝ I experience clitoral orgasms in many different forms. It all depends on the duration of the sex or masturbation session and the tools that are used. When I'm alone, it's faster and shorter. With a vibrator it's pure pleasure from the get go, but the orgasm—even though it's a big, intense eruption—will be brief. When my partner does the fingering it takes at least 10 minutes before it really starts tingling down there. Depending on how aroused I am, it can take another 5 to 10 minutes before I come. When I finally go over the edge, I feel waves of pleasure. They wash over me, basically, to the rhythm of my vagina's contractions. The world appears to come to a standstill for a moment. My body will be writhing and I'll be shuddering for a few more seconds. ❞

Eva (27)

What is it?

Unlike the penis, the clitoris is a bit hidden away. If you've never seen your own clitoris, it's high time to start exploring. Grab a mirror and stick it between your legs. Say hello to your vulva. Go on, they don't bite. . . . Your little bud is covered by a hood. If you spread your labia with two fingers, you'll see it. The visible part of the clitoris is known as the "glans." Every clitoris looks different. It can be anywhere between one-eighth and three-eighths of an inch (three and eight mm) in size. Arousal causes blood to flow to your clitoris and the internal erectile tissue to grow. This doesn't just make penetration feel good, but the swollen tissues also act as airbags, so your partner's thrusting isn't painful.

Quickie

For AFABs, the clitoris has no fewer than 8,000 nerve endings, twice as many as the glans penis. But, unfortunately, that doesn't necessarily entail coming better, faster, or more easily.

How to get there?
THE BUILD-UP

You can achieve a clitoral orgasm by stimulating the clitoris with fingers, tongue, or a sex toy. Don't immediately descend on that clit though—it's too intense, and for some people it's even painful. Instead, slowly build the tension. The more turned-on you are, the greater the release and the more intense your happy ending. Start at what are the least sensitive places for you. These could include the neck, throat, earlobes, and mouth. Then take it a step further and target the more sensitive spots like your breasts, nipples, and buttocks. Keep going like this until you arrive at your biggest pleasure organ, the clitoris.

TEASING IS PLEASING

Teasing (solo or by a partner) will leave you wanting more. Gradually speed things up. Once you're wet or have lubricated enough, you can stroke the labia or clitoris every now and then. Using fingers or a toy, trace circles around your labia and occasionally touch the clit. Do it just often enough to give your body a taste of what's to come. If it's something you like, you can massage your breasts or thighs at the same time. Keep going until you're crazy with lust. Only then do you get to release yourself from your heavenly suffering and focus fully on that hotspot.

TRACING FIGURES

Circles, triangles, straight lines . . . or the entire alphabet. What figures you trace between your labia is entirely up to you. One thing's for sure: There's plenty to discover. Try every trick to find out what works best for you.

Many people find direct contact with the clitoris too intense. Luckily there are some easy techniques to take the pressure off. Here's how.

1. Place your index and middle finger to the left and right of your inner labia. If you bring them together, you should feel your clitoris. Move your fingers in circles, up and down, or left to right. The stimulation will be pleasant, but not direct.

2. Place one or two fingers on the clitoral hood. Gently press it down over the glans of your clit and back up again. To avoid touching the actual clitoris make sure your finger doesn't slip.

3. Stimulate your clitoris over your underwear. The little piece of fabric will take the edge off things. But do remember to make sure that your labia is wet—naturally or with a bit of store-bought lubricant—or else it might still feel a bit rough.

Is a direct, hands-on approach not an issue for you? In that case you can deploy these dexterous techniques.

1. Place two or three outstretched fingers on your clitoris and move them around in big ovals. Your fingers don't just touch your clit, but your labia, too.

2. Place a finger directly on your clitoris and trace tiny circles while applying some gentle pressure. Your finger doesn't leave your clit.

3. Do the same as above, but this time move your finger. Start your circles at the hood and touch the clitoris, but also a little bit of the surrounding area, too.

4. Not a fan of circles? Caress up and down between your urethra and your clitoris. Explore what feels best for you: applying more pressure on the way there or on the way back.

SLOWLY DOES IT

Climaxing is not a race to the finish line. Are you feeling it? Are the technique, pressure, speed, and rhythm just right? Don't be tempted to go harder and faster right away. It's usually counterproductive. Maintain your technique and very slowly speed things up. Keep breathing calmly, focus on the sensation, relax your body, clear your head of worries and fill it with fantasy—and let the orgasm last and last.

Vaginal orgasm

66 My boyfriend's on top, penetrating me, not too gentle and not too hard either. My vagina is becoming more and more sensitive. I can tell from his breathing that he's close to orgasm. The suspense of his imminent climax makes me even more receptive and when he starts thrusting deeper and harder we come at the same time. My vagina contracts around his penis and I feel my whole body relax. The orgasm is wonderful and lasts a long time, but it does feel more muted than a clitoral climax. 99

Fiona (28)

What is it?
As we said, only 10 to 20 percent of women report coming via penetration alone. And by that we mean without additional stim-ulation of the external clitoris. Not everyone can achieve this. It

depends on your anatomy. The closer the erectile tissue of your internal clitoris is to your vagina, the greater the chance that you can come through penetration. But there are some useful tricks and moves that may help you to tick that elusive vaginal orgasm off your bucket list.

How to get there
GIRTH IS BETTER THAN LENGTH

Some of us sometimes like to gossip about the length of our new flame's penis, but we really ought to be asking about girth! Yep, it's girth you should consider when it comes to vaginal stimulation. An extra-long penis can jostle the cervix or otherwise be uncomfortable . . . and what's the point of that? For AFABs, the opening of the vagina and the first four inches are far more sensitive than the end of the vagina, as they have the most nerve endings. About one to two inches in is the G-spot (more about this later), and up to about four inches in, the swollen clitoris can still be stimulated. So the thicker the instrument of love, the better it'll entertain.

SHALLOW

Make sure that—as always—you're thoroughly warmed up before you head toward the V-zone. Are you fully aroused (and especially: wet)? Start massaging your clitoris, so the internal part becomes engorged. Stop before you come and then focus on your vagina. Massage the entrance slowly and with a slight pressure. Does this leave you wanting more? Insert one finger and trace small circles. Now step up both the pace and the pressure. Note: You don't need deep thrusts to achieve a vaginal orgasm. Short, slow thrusts with your partner pulling all the way out of your vagina are best for stimulating the nerves. A penis can do this, but so can a dildo or two or more fingers. Try them all and see what works best for you!

IN POSITION

Few sexual positions (without additional manual or oral stimulation) minister to the clitoris directly. There's really only one that truly serves the pleasure bud, and that's the CAT position (see page 153 for the illustration). Although it will leave you purring, it's got nothing to do with cats. CAT stands for Coital Alignment Technique. It's like missionary, but different, and much more enjoyable. Your partner lies fairly high above you, with their chest at your shoulder height. You place your legs at a 45-degree angle. Instead of thrusting, your partner moves their hips in a circular motion. It's crucial that their pubic bone makes maximum contact with your clitoris. With this technique both the opening of the vagina and the clitoris receive plenty of stimulation. Once the two of you have mastered this, you need to keep going. Focus on the chafing sensation, breathe in and out, and surrender. It takes a bit of practice, but after that it's pure pleasure.

A HELPING HAND

Are you close to coming, but just can't get beyond the point of no return? A bit of assistance is fine as far as we're concerned. Place an index finger on the glans of your clitoris, apply moderate pressure, and gently trace circles or rhythmically tap on or around your clit. This little extra can push you over the edge. Coming through simultaneous stimulation of two sexual zones is known as a mixed orgasm. But who knows, if you practice enough you may eventually manage it without help from the glans stimulation.

Anal orgasm

❝ We wanted to explore the anus as an erogenous zone. He fingered the outside of my 'back door' and with his other hand he massaged my buttocks. He left my vagina alone. Suddenly I felt these sensations that were very similar to a G-spot orgasm washing over me. The waves of pleasure kept coming. Longer than a clitoral orgasm, which is more of an explosive thing for me. It felt like a very fun and naughty orgasm. Since that first time it's also been really easy to achieve. **❞**

Maureen (32)

What is it?

Climaxing via anal sex? I understand if you're skeptical. From reproduction's point of view, your back door isn't "made" for sex. So how are you supposed to come via anal play? Thankfully, just about anything is possible in the wonderful world that is sex. If you think that the anus is no more than an exit, think again. There really is such a thing as an anal orgasm. The opening is surrounded by lots of extremely sensitive nerve endings, which makes the right kind of touch so delicious. It's also right next to your vagina and connected to your clitoris. As Samantha Jones put it so eloquently in *Sex and the City*, "With the right guy and the right lubricant . . . it's fabulous." Though she was mistaken about one thing: You don't necessarily need a "guy" to achieve it!

Lara: So you still haven't told me. What do you think counts as sex?
Dana: I don't know. Having an orgasm.
Lara: Well, if that was the case, that would mean thousands of women who are married with children have never had sex.

Lara Perkins and Dana Fairbanks
in *The L Word*

This Big O often feels a bit different from the one achieved through direct clitoral stimulation. The experience can be more intense and deeply sensual. Some lucky people can come through butt sex alone, while others need additional clitoral and/or vaginal stimulation to reach a climax. We'll count this as an anal orgasm, too. Research has shown that engaging in anal play may lead to more frequent happy endings, period. For 94 percent of the women in one 2015 study from the National Survey of Sexual Health and Behavior, it was part of a magic combination for an awesome climax.

> ## *Quickie*
> **Over the years anal sex has become more and more popular. In a 2010 study from The Journal of Sexual Medicine, 40 percent of women between the ages of 20 and 24 reported trying it, up from just 16 percent in the early 1990s.**

How to get there

An anal orgasm can be achieved through (duh) anal sex: both rimming (using the tongue to stimulate the anus) and penetration with one or more fingers, a penis, or a sex toy.

LUBRICANT

Porn creates the illusion that a penis can simply slide one-two-three into your back door. Nope! Unlike your vagina, the anus doesn't self-lubricate to ease penetration. So add this to your shopping list: an XL tube of silicone lube. The silicone variant doesn't dry up and isn't sticky. Numbing anal lubes also exist, but they aren't recommended. They can inhibit your ability to feel pain, and pain is your body telling you important information!

PREPARATION IS EVERYTHING

One of the most common—and biggest—fear people have is that their stool will come out during anal sex. Unless you're suffering from a terrible bout of diarrhea or you're having really rough and reckless sex, this won't happen. But it's wise to empty your bowels before you get it on. Then wash thoroughly for the necessary hygiene. For your own peace of mind, you can put a towel under your butt. An anal douche is another option, but not one that we recommend. Frequent use can upset your bowel function.

Speaking of hygiene: Beware of going from A to V. We don't want to spoil the fun, but your anus is a source of bacteria. Go from vaginal sex to anal sex, but never the other way around. Are you determined to end the sex at V? Then make sure your partner uses a condom during anal (or a dental dam). Remove it (and put on a new one if necessary) before you have vaginal sex again.

TURNED ON

Anal doesn't lend itself to a "quickie." It calls for serious preparation. It's also super important that you're really aroused. You need to be able to fully relax and surrender to your partner. Long "foreplay" is an absolute must. Make sure you don't come because then your pelvic floor muscles will contract again, which makes anal sex much harder.

STEP BY STEP

Start by massaging the anus to get used to the touch. Then slowly and carefully insert a finger or a slender butt plug. Coat it generously with silicone or anal lube. Fight the impulse to contract your muscles by calmly breathing in and out. Rub your clitoris to turn yourself on and to help you to relax.

If all this goes smoothly, you can take it a bit further: two fingers or a slightly bigger butt plug. You can leave it at that of course. But if you want something a little bigger, you can switch to the penis, dildo, or a butt plug in a larger size. Some people prefer a (non-vibrating) butt plug. Unlike a penis or dildo that goes up and down, the toy provides a subtle stimulus.

POSITIONS

The positions you go for are the key to good anal sex. You can't be quite so wild as you might be during "regular" sex. Being on top is out of the question for many people. For beginners, spooning is a comfortable position. It stops your partner from going too deep or too fast. They're doing the moving, but you're in control. Missionary is another good option, because you can see each other's faces and communicate better. It's also a bit more intimate and you can reach your clitoris more easily. Get used to the sensation first before you start experimenting with other positions.

CLEAR COMMUNICATION

Trust, relaxation, and communication are essential for pain-free and pleasurable anal play. Ask your bed partner to tell you, step by step, what they're going to do, and indicate clearly when you're ready for more and especially if and when you need a break. Does it hurt? In that case, your preparations may have fallen short. Maybe you're too tense, your sphincter isn't relaxed enough, your partner is going at it a bit too rough, and/or you've skimped on the lube. Again: Take your time.

Nipple orgasm

66 My then partner was a skilled tantric sex practitioner. Thanks to yoni (vaginal) massage, body massage, and breathing techniques my entire body was in a state of ecstasy. I felt at one with my partner, my surroundings, and the universe. As she was kissing, sucking, and licking my nipples, she placed her hand gently on my stomach. After a while, I erupted into an orgasm that made my whole body shudder. My clitoris, vagina, legs, torso, arms . . . seriously, my whole body was shuddering and tingling. I saw stars; it lasted for minutes. Wow! 99

Elly (49)

What is it?

Most people can be divided into two camps: Those who love a bit of nipple play and those who can't stand having their nipples and/ or breasts fondled. If you're in the first group you might like to find out whether you can have a nipple orgasm. Yup, there is such a thing! The nerves in nipples are connected to the brain and cli- toris. That means that stimulation of the 800 nerve endings in nipples can be felt in your private parts. It's often used as a little something to complement penetration or oral sex, but with the right technique it *is* possible to climax through nipple stimulation alone.

A nipple orgasm feels totally different from a "regular" one; in fact, everyone tends to experience it in their own way. Unlike a clitoral orgasm, it usually doesn't culminate in a peak. The pleasure sweeps through your body in waves or in spurts. But this, too, counts as coming. Some people even experience an actual full-blown climax during a nipple orgasm.

How to get there

Arousal is a must for any orgasm. Even more so for a nipple orgasm. A rich imagination and strong mindset will do the rest.

A JOURNEY OF DISCOVERY

Lots of people feel a bit funny about touching their breasts. Are you one of them? Then it's high time you got to know your boobies. Think of them as your bosom buddies. Study them—without a bra—in the mirror and massage, squeeze, and push them around. Lean forward, backward, or stand on your head if you like. It may be a silly sight, but it will help you to grow more used to your breasts.

> ## Quickie
> **Did you know that your nipples tend to become extra sensitive around ovulation? That's the moment to discover the nipple orgasm.**

GETTING INTO IT

Is nipple play totally new to you? Find out—either solo or with a bed partner—what you enjoy. Play with your breasts during masturbation or when you're being fingered, eaten out, or penetrated. Or let your partner get to work on your nipples with their fingers or tongue. That way you get used to the idea and you'll associate stimulation of your breasts and nipples with coming. With each masturbation session or bout of sex you can gradually shift attention from the clit to your nipples until you're only pampering your breasts and nipples.

EROTIC MASSAGE

As with any other orgasm, you need to build up to it slowly. Don't descend on those nips right away, but start by caressing, massaging, and kneading your breasts and/or the surrounding area. Use a bit of lube or massage oil. Push your nipples in, roll them between your thumb and index fingers, squeeze them. . . . Try it all and note when you feel something stirring in your nether regions.

That's how you know you're on the right track. Stick to this technique and slowly increase the tempo. Let your imagination run wild and focus on the sensation. Start by taking slow, deep breaths and speed up your breathing as you approach your climax. Rhythmically contracting and relaxing your pelvic floor can also help to push you over the edge.

DELEGATE

Once you know what turns you on, you can share it with your sex partner. Give clear instructions. If you're uncomfortable doing this during sex, explain what you like before you start. Other than that, short and sharp "orders" like "harder," "gentler," "more pressure," and "less pressure" do the trick.

Quickie

Some people have such sensitive nipples that they can have an orgasm-like sensation while breastfeeding. If it sounds weird, don't be ashamed! The reaction is more hormonal than sexual: Breastfeeding releases oxytocin, which produces the orgasm-like sensation.

Zone orgasm

66 The soles of my feet are extremely sensitive. Prolonged touch can bring me to orgasm. When my partner runs an ice cube along the soles of my feet, I experience this really intense sensation throughout my body. It's a total *wow!* 99

Jasmine (43)

What is it?

One step beyond the nipple orgasm we find the zone orgasm. Erogenous zones are located all over your body. We all know the effect of touching the clitoris, vagina, and nipples, but the earlobes, throat, neck, soles of the feet, buttocks, thighs, and navel are erogenous, too. Such sweet spots are personal to you. While some go wild for a head massage, others are in seventh heaven when someone sucks on their little toe. Spanking, sucking on the inner thighs, or a tongue in the navel—the possibilities are endless, and to each their own. With the right timing, mindset, and technique it's possible to turn these stimuli into an orgasm: It's known as a zone orgasm. It takes a lot of practice and concentration, but it's definitely doable.

How to get there?

SET THE MOOD

Any bout of sex, solo or otherwise, can be enhanced by mood makers, but with something as challenging as a zone orgasm it's an absolute must. Go overboard with reed diffusers, body mists, dimmed lighting, candles, crisp white sheets, your favorite comfy clothes, massage oil, and some sultry tunes. The works. More is more in this case. And don't forget to put that eternal mood breaker—your cell phone—on silent and leave it somewhere out of reach and out of sight.

MINDFUL MINDSET

It's a lot harder to reach orgasms that don't involve direct or indirect stimulation of your clit. They require more practice and you need to be more relaxed, confident, and imaginative. Take the time to discover all of your happy places. It could take up to an hour before you start to feel something.

NEXT-LEVEL MASSAGE

You don't technically achieve a zone orgasm by combining "manual work," oral sex, or penetration with something like nibbling an earlobe. That's all well and good, but for a zone climax you focus on just one single area. You can start by massaging multiple places to light your fire, but the ultimate aim is to ignite a single erogenous zone until you explode with pleasure. Use a drop of lube or a fragrant massage oil to enhance the experience. Caress, massage, knead, and squeeze your body all over until you discover the contact you like best.

CHANGE IT UP
A touch can feel totally different depending on whether you're sitting or lying down. Press your feet together, lean them against the wall, or throw your legs behind your head. Experimentation is allowed—no, mandatory! And remember: Being super chill and confident is what matters most.

G-spot orgasm

❝ We start with foreplay to make sure I'm really aroused. Then we move on to penetration for a while. Next, she sits down beside me and seems to use all the strength in her forearms to touch my G-spot in a very specific way. She pushes and presses firm and fast. As a result, I experience a huge sense of release that can go on and on and on. And it's become quite normal for me to squirt. It's phenomenal! **❞**

Anne (38)

What is it?

The Atlantis among orgasms: the G-spot. The debate has been raging for dozens of years: Does it exist or not? You may want to sit down for this. Yes, it exists. But maybe not in the way it's often described or talked about. "It's not a separate organ, but the back of the clitoris and the erectile tissue of the urethra, which is wedged between the anterior vaginal wall and the back of the clitoris," explains sexologist Ellen Laan. When you're massively turned on, this Gräfenberg spot swells up. The right technique can lead to a really intense orgasm. Although you're indirectly stimulating the clit, a G-spot orgasm feels completely different from a clitoral one. For post-op trans people, the G-spot is their prostate. Most people don't experience a peak, but very deep and powerful waves of pleasure.

Squirting

G-spot stimulation can trigger a squirting orgasm. Forget what you often see in porn films, it doesn't look like a bottle of champagne being uncorked. If you suddenly become extremely wet during G-spot stimulation, it means you've squirted. Although some people squirt like a drinking fountain, most don't. It's good to know that the squirting itself doesn't give any extra pleasure. The orgasm is just as good without the splashing.

How to get there

A voyage of discovery to your G-spot: You can travel solo or with a partner. Experience tells us that the second is easier, as you can lie back and totally relax. It's just that little bit less difficult for another person to reach. If you do decide to go it alone, we suggest you get a G-spot toy.

Start by stimulating your clit. This boosts the blood flow to your vagina and engorges your G-spot. The more aroused you are, the better the stimulation feels. Are you on the verge? Insert two fingers into your vagina and go in search of a "spongy" bit some one-and-a-half to two inches inside the vagina. Got it? Use your two fingers to make a "come here" gesture and apply pressure to the spot. But ignore what you've seen in porn—they go at it with far too much gusto. Slowly building your rhythm and speed is key. A gentle rhythm and firm pressure are often intense enough. Are you breathing faster and is the sensation spreading throughout your lower abdomen? Step up the pace, mind your breathing, and relax.

The swelling puts pressure on your bladder. You feel as if you need to pee, but you can ignore that. When you relax your pelvic floor muscles and fully surrender, you may start squirting. No luck? No worries. For extra stimulation, you can press your thumb against the clitoris and gently trace circles. Scale this back every time you experiment until you can do it without! Yes, you can!

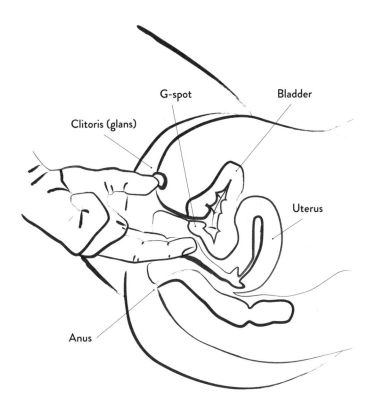

G-spot

Bladder

Clitoris (glans)

Uterus

Anus

Squirting = peeing?

A frequently asked question about squirting is this: What's coming out? Is it urine? Some scientists reckon it is, others disagree. The fluid doesn't look like pee. It's not yellow and doesn't smell or taste like urine. Then what is it? A mixture of different juices, so to speak. For AFABs, it's made up of the ejaculate from the Skene's gland, vaginal self-lubrication fluid, secretion from the uterus, and, for the rest, mostly diluted urine. The pee that's produced during stimulation of the G-spot is more watery and, because it's mixed with other discharge, both its color and smell change. It's not entirely clear whether you squirt from your bladder or your vagina. Because the squirting liquid contains prostate fluid, some sex scientists say that it must come from the Skene's glands. Then again, anatomically speaking, only the bladder can produce this amount of fluid. The fuller your bladder when you come squirting, the greater the chance that it looks, smells, and tastes of urine. Having sex on a full bladder isn't a good idea anyway, so we recommend you do a number one before you get going.

A-spot orgasm

❝ I can only experience an A-spot orgasm via deep, steady penetration. Mostly in missionary with my legs behind my neck [the Viennese oyster]. The trick is that he goes in really deep, stays there, and goes a bit further with each thrust. It's an orgasm that knocks me out. . . . It gives me an out-of-body experience and it leaves me on a high. I really need time to recover afterward. ❞

Katrina (29)

What is it?

The A-spot is a well-kept secret. It's rarely spoken or written about, despite its discovery in 1994 by a Malaysian doctor. In the course of his research, he came across an extremely sensitive zone deep inside the vagina. The A-spot, also known as the anterior fornix, is situated along the front vaginal wall and close to the cervix for AFABs. For post-op trans people, this same spot is the seminal vesicles.

The A-spot is an extension of the clitoris, but like many of the other orgasms in this chapter the sensation is very different. You can feel it from head to toe. It can give you something akin to an out-of-body experience. Sounds good, don't you think? Here's another benefit: Whereas the clitoris is soon "overcome" by all the attention, you can keep stimulating the A-spot . . . even after an orgasm.

But please take note! The A-spot is extremely sensitive. Some people find prolonged stimulation too intense. So we'll repeat our mantra: Take it easy, take your time, and keep practicing.

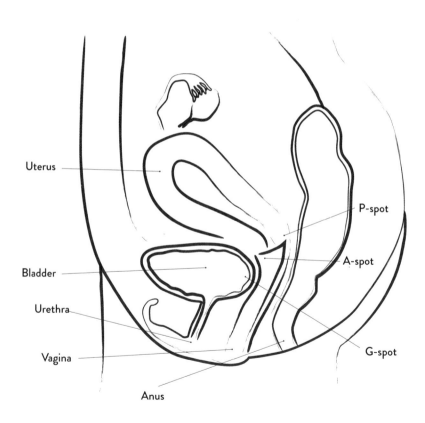

Uterus

P-spot

A-spot

Bladder

Urethra

Vagina

G-spot

Anus

How to get there

AROUSAL IS KEY

We can't stress this enough: a body in a state of total arousal is essential if you want to come. So, too, for the A-spot orgasm. Because this hotspot is close to the ultrasensitive cervix (if you have one), your vagina has to be totally ready (read: wet, relaxed, and distended) before you jump into action. If it's not, trying to find your anterior fornix can be painful.

ON THE HUNT

Finding the A-spot is something for advanced learners. The spot is literally out of reach. You need a partner with long fingers. A long and slender sex toy with a curved tip is also effective. A penis is often too short and doesn't have the right shape to hit the spot. Lean against the headboard or wall in a slouching position with your knees pulled up. Insert your tool of choice deep into your vagina. Explore the front of the cervix in search of a sensitive spot the size of a quarter. You'll know when you've found it.

WARMING UP

Patience is a virtue. It can take a while before you experience the A-spot thrill. After the necessary "foreplay" to warm up, you can gently massage the A-spot for twenty to thirty minutes. Lightly press against the front wall using a circular motion. Once you're into the groove, you can increase the pressure a bit. But maintain the same technique and pace throughout—don't go too hard or thrust into it. Take deep breaths in and out, relax your body, and focus on the sensation. Close your eyes if you prefer.

Cervical orgasm

" It's a feeling like no other. So primal, so womanly, so loving! It came about after lengthy stimulation with his fingers—sometimes tender, sometimes firm—of my vagina and cervix. I was taking deep and slow breaths from my stomach. We never took our eyes off each other. The orgasm began gently and the tingling sensation throughout my body lasted for what felt like an hour. It wasn't a peak orgasm, but deliciously long and deep. Like it should be. **"**

Robin (44)

What is it?

Many AFABs know how sensitive the uterus and especially the cervix can be. Think of menstrual cramps, an IUD insertion, or childbirth. . . . But in addition to pain, the uterus can also be a source of wonderful feelings. The uterine nerve pathway—known as the hypogastric plexus—is connected to the vagina. The right stimulation of this hotspot can lead to a divine climax. The cervical orgasm is also known as the P-spot orgasm, the P standing for post fornix (it's situated opposite the A-spot). But please note: Cervical stimulation may not be your cup of tea. The cervix is the barrier to the uterus and can be very sensitive—in the negative sense of the word. Some people experience joy, others mostly pain.

Quickie

Prostate owners have a P-spot, too. Massage it during a hand job, blowjob, or full-on sex to give them a more intense orgasm. Insert your index finger some two inches into the rectum, find the walnut-sized knob (the prostate), and stimulate it with a gentle "come here" motion.

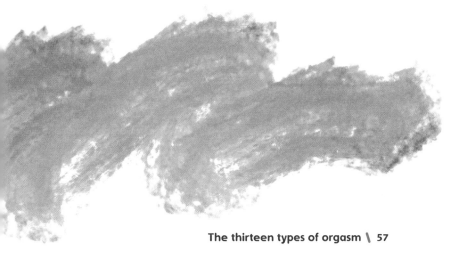

How to get there

PREPARATION

This orgasm is incredibly intense, so the right preparation is absolutely vital. Every body responds differently to cervical stimulation, so take your time to discover what does and doesn't work for you. Start by making sure that your body is completely relaxed. Lie down flat on your back and place your hands on your abdomen. Breathe in and out and concentrate on your center. What are you feeling? Focus on your body and not on your mind. Let go of any negative emotions. Keep doing this until you feel as light as a feather.

> ## Quickie
> **Did you know that in tantric sex, tension is thought to be stored in the uterus?**

CERVICAL MASSAGE

Maximizing your arousal is the next step. Like the A-spot, your cervix is more open to stimulation when you're thoroughly limbered up. Proceed carefully. Begin with a gentle cervical massage. If either your fingers or those of your lover are too short, you can use a long dildo. Start by slowly tracing circles around your cervix to get used to the sensation. Then try applying gentle pressure or slide from side to side. Keep breathing deeply and calmly while relaxing your body and mind and opening yourself up to the unfamiliar. Once you get going, you can slowly increase the pressure. But please note: only the pressure, not the pace. Your cervix isn't too pleased with quick and sudden movements. Tip: Massaging your cervix for a half hour is no luxury. This organ calls for just that little bit more patience than your clitoris. But you know what they say: Good things come to those who wait.

Quickie

Your cervix is particularly irritable around the times of menstruation and ovulation. That's why a massage can feel very different from one attempt to the next. Is it not doing anything for you? Try again the following week!

CALLING THE SHOTS

Are you exploring with a partner? Always communicate. You're in control. You should be the one telling them what to do and how to do it.

Delivery orgasm

It may be hard to believe, but it's true! It's possible to (consciously or not) reach a climax while giving birth to a baby. During the delivery the body produces the happy hormones endorphin and oxytocin. Add to this the fact that the womb contracts and pushes the baby's head up against the clitoris and the result can sometimes be a wonderful feeling. While things may get awkward in the delivery room, it does relieve the pain of the contractions. If you like the sound of that, sorry to disappoint you, but it is, unsurprisingly, rare: It happens in just 0.3 percent of births.

U-spot orgasm

❝ To relax, I start by receiving a massage or massaging myself. I need to be really aroused before I can work toward a U-spot orgasm. With a finger I'll gently caress or stroke the area. Aside from stroking, a kind of tapping motion can be quite nice, too. I maintain the tempo and intensity. After a while I can feel the entire area contract. I keep going, using the same technique. And then I feel an amazing energy course through my body. **❞**

Amy (43)

What is it?

The clitoris is purely for pleasure, the vagina for baby making *and* pleasure. And the urethra . . . ? Just for emptying your bladder? Wrong! When we're talking about the urethra, we often think only of relieving ourselves, but your pee hole is capable of so much more. Introducing the U-spot orgasm.

The spot is located between the clitoris and the vaginal opening and is invisible to the naked eye. While the urethra can rightly call itself an erogenous zone, as it's surrounded by nerve endings on three sides, the U-spot isn't the urethra itself, but the soft tissue around it. When you rub it, it starts swelling up. After a while, you'll experience a delightful sensation. With the right moves you can reach a climax.

How to get there
SAFETY FIRST

The U-spot and your urethra are extremely sensitive, so always be gentle. The last thing you want is small tears that could become infected. That's why a moist environment is a must. The glands inside your inner labia self-lubricate. But an extra drop of lube doesn't hurt either.

FINGERWORK

A U-spot orgasm may seem challenging, but here's a stroke of luck. One type of stimulation works particularly well: circular motions. Use your index finger to trace circles around your urethra. Start slowly and be mindful of your body's response. Is there no tingling yet? Increase both pace and pressure a tiny bit. Try this for another 5 minutes and continue like this until you find out what works best for you. Keep going until you experience a peak.

ORAL

Your fingers are ideal tools for discovering your U-spot, but some people prefer a tongue. For this you obviously need a partner. Ask them to gently trace circles around your urethra opening with a pointy tongue. Explore together what rhythm, intensity, and pressure work for you both.

Are you nearly-nearly-nearly there, but can't quite get over the edge to orgasm? You can help things along by letting a (non-vibrating) dildo or finger rest inside your vagina.

Throat orgasm

“ While deep throating I've been surprised by the occasional climax. It really felt like coming. He could go a lot deeper without it hurting, my throat constricted, and my vagina contracted and became really wet. At that moment it really felt as if my throat and vagina were connected. ”

Carly (41)

What is it?

We can hear you thinking: This has got to be a joke. But no, strangely enough the throat orgasm isn't the brainchild of men aimed at making deep throating popular among women. People really can experience a throat orgasm. Science has shown that a nerve inside your throat is connected to your cervix. A throat orgasm revolves around a spot that's located very deep inside the throat, at the opening, right behind your windpipe. To stimulate that spot, you need to become an expert deep throater. When you achieve it, your throat starts glowing while a wave of lust and pleasure surges through your body. It's not for everyone though. Are you not open to it? Then don't even try it. You only reach an orgasm if you let yourself. Are blowjobs in general not your thing? Then skip the next couple of pages.

The throat orgasm was discovered by accident. It is particularly popular in the tantric sex community, because the throat is a chakra (or energy point in the body) and symbolizes creativity, innovation, and expression. So you might even achieve a creative breakthrough after a throat orgasm!

Quickie
Deep throating is the blowing technique in which the penis goes all the way inside the blower's mouth—or at least as much as humanly possible. The point is that it at least goes deep into the throat.

How to get there
TRUST
Not 90 percent or 99.9999 percent, but 100 percent: Exploring a throat orgasm all comes down to trusting each other. Blowjobs put you in a vulnerable position at the best of times, and taking the whole of a penis into your mouth is the most extreme expression of this. The ball is in your court at all times. Clear communi-

cation is vital. Because you can't talk you'll have to agree on signals beforehand.

MIND-BLOWING HEAD

Is oral sex something you do 1) especially for your partner,
2) always reluctantly, or 3) something you enjoy, too? Don't
view a blowjob as a chore, but an intimate gift you can share
with your partner. Then you will be able to give it your all fully
and be mentally prepared to discover the throat orgasm. The
remarkable thing about the throat orgasm, compared to some
of the other orgasms, is that you both experience pleasure at
the same time when it's happening.

IN POSITION

Make yourself more comfortable by lying on your back with your
head over the edge of the bed. In this position the gag reflex is
less acute. This way your partner will also find it easy to slide into
your throat. It's up to you whether you want to move your head
or have them thrust. Do you feel more comfortable in a different
position? Then start there. Above all, you need to be able to relax.

PRACTICE MAKES PERFECT

Deep throating like a porn star isn't something you'll pull off at
your first attempt. You can only learn through lots and lots of
practice. Some people will find it easier than others. The more
sensitive your gag reflex, the trickier it's going to be. Train your-

self by taking your partner a bit further into your throat each time. To achieve a throat orgasm, the penis will have to linger there for a while. Let them make circular movements or bob gently up and down. It all hinges on remaining calm and taking deep, steady breaths. It helps if you flare your nostrils as wide as possible. Some people like to close their eyes, so they can focus better.

Mental orgasm

❝ I imagine being pursued by an animal, and I'm running away from him. When he catches up with me, I feel a mixture of fear and excitement. He overpowers me and bites my neck. Being wanted, someone actively chasing me after I tell him I'm his—this excites me so much that my body responds. It starts prickling and tingling. Blood flows to my labia and they start throbbing. At the imaginary moment when he enters me, I feel my clitoris pulsate and I wake from my daydream with a sharp, but wonderful peak. ❞

Janine (33)

What is it?

Coming without being touched: It. Is. Possible. From our teenage years it's drummed into us that having a climax is a question of the hottest position, the best technique, and an experienced lover. All physical requirements. But ultimately, an orgasm depends on what's happening inside your head: An orgasm is all between the ears.

A mental orgasm or *mindgasm* is a climax that you generate purely on the strength of your thoughts. It's the very definition of hands-free coming. The sensation is different for everyone, but it's not unlike a clitoral or a G-spot orgasm. The more you practice, the more skilled you become, and the easier you can achieve this peak orgasm.

> ## Quickie
> **Our brain is our most powerful sex organ. No mental excitement = no physical excitement.**

How to get there
FREE YOUR MIND AND THE REST WILL FOLLOW

A mindgasm requires total concentration and relaxation. You know how easily your mind can flutter from one thought to the next. So start meditating. Install a meditation app on your phone and for a week spend fifteen minutes every day training yourself to empty your head.

IN POSITION
Once you master this skill, you can start exploring your mental orgasm. Create a nice atmosphere in your room. Lie down on a freshly made, soft bed. Loosen up your limbs for a minute or so and place your arms beside your body. Bend your knees so your vagina can "breathe."

FEEL YOUR FANTASY
A lively imagination will come in handy now. But even if you're not much of a dreamer you can still achieve a mental orgasm. Everyone has a sexual fantasy that turns them on. Maybe it's erotic role play that gets you going, or else a particular person you'd like to share a bed with. Or think of a certain sex position—or positions—that gets you all fired up. Play out that fantasy in your head. Imagine in minute detail what's happening in your fantasy world and what it might feel like. Focus on the subtle tingling in your body and try to enhance it by diving even deeper into your imaginary world.

FAKE IT TILL YOU MAKE IT
But fantasy alone won't get you there. You may not be touching your body, but that doesn't mean you can't move. The idea is simple: You're going to simulate an orgasm with your mind. Take deep breaths in and out, rhythmically move your butt and pelvis up and

down, engage your pelvic floor and relax it again. Try a push and pull motion with your pelvic muscles and try to summon the physical feeling you have in your vagina when you come. Find your sexy rhythm and stick to it. The closer you get to your climax, the faster your breathing and movements become.

"I can actually mentally give myself an orgasm. You know, sense memory is quite powerful."

Lady Gaga in *New York Magazine*

THINK: ORGASM

Now is the time to let the power of the mind take over. Think "I'm awesome," "I'm sexy," and "I'm gorgeous." Your thoughts about yourself will have an immediate impact on your body. You'll automatically start thinking, "I'm coming, I'm coming." Have faith, believe that your thoughts can become reality. Relax and become one with your body. Let your body respond to your fantasy images. Try to feel the orgasm, breathe faster, move your pelvis to the rhythm, and surrender.

TAKE IT EASY

Is it not happening? Don't be discouraged if you don't feel something right away. Linking your mind and your vagina is a slow and challenging process. Keep experimenting and believing in yourself.

> ### *Quickie*
> **It's easier to achieve a mental orgasm when you're already spontaneously aroused. That way, you have a head start—and you can use less mental energy to get you to the climax.**

Coregasm

❝ The first time it happened I was in high school. I was running laps when I felt a glowing sensation in my groin. It was a shock, because I wasn't familiar with the feeling of an orgasm. But I figured it felt pretty good, so I carried on running. At some point I reached a climax. Although the feeling was new to me, I realized that it was something intimate. **❞**

Nora (37)

What is it?

Sex is like sports. You work up a sweat and if you've done your best you may well be sore the following morning. But it also works the other way around: Sports can be sexy, too. A US study from 2014 found that one in ten women has had a happy ending doing sports. And no, they weren't chafing on their bicycle seat or being naughty and sitting on a vibration plate. During a coregasm, you're taken by surprise while exercising. Sexual stimulation doesn't come into it. Then how is it possible, you ask? "Many women [sic] need a build-up of tension in their legs before they can reach an orgasm," sex therapist Victoria Zdrok explains. "When an exercising woman produces extra endorphins and dopamine, substances needed for an orgasm, and she flexes the muscles in her abdomen, the clitoris may be indirectly stimulated."

How to get there?

Unfortunately there are no manuals on how to achieve a coregasm. It just happens. But you can create the right conditions for it. Exercises that train the lower abdominals, in particular, get the clitoris going. The sensation is most powerful when the legs are relaxed and the stomach muscles flexed. Think of abdominal exercises and weight training.

Multiple orgasm

66 It's not unusual for me to have multiple, successive orgasms. Quite the opposite: I often can't stop at one. I can achieve it via certain positions, but also with a toy. Sometimes there are short pauses between the climaxes, sometimes it's one long series of orgasms. It's an intense and full body experience: trembling legs, muscle spasms, and squirting. But it's incredibly exhausting. Afterward, my muscles ache and I'll be hypersensitive to the point of pain. However great it may sound . . . it's not always pleasurable. 99

Martha (53)

What is it?

What's better than one orgasm? How about two or three or . . . it's known as a multiple orgasm. Don't worry if you can "only" come once or if you're having trouble with round one. You're not alone. A double or triple orgasm is something few can pull off, but it's not impossible. Try it solo or with a "helping hand" using the following techniques.

How to get there
A BRIEF PAUSE

The clitoris will often be too sensitive after round one to immediately resume. Direct touch is usually too intense, causing your body to "convulse." In fact, it can hurt. So take a moment to catch your breath after your first climax.

> ## Quickie
> **Extra lube will make the friction on your clitoris less intense.**

VARIETY IS THE SPICE OF LIFE

Start round two by stimulating erogenous zones other than your clit. Think of the breasts, earlobes, buttocks, thighs, or neck. Whatever floats your boat. It allows you to slowly restart your engine and to give your oversensitive clitoris a break. After five to ten minutes (or however long it takes you personally!) you can focus on your pleasure bud again. Take a totally different approach this time. Use different techniques (see clitoral orgasm, page 29): three fingers instead of one, your nondominant hand, or assume a different position (see chaper 6). Usually these three approaches are especially effective: slowing down, easing up on the pressure, and focusing less on the clit.

Try switching to another kind of orgasm. Have you just come after a clitoral orgasm? Then why not try a G-spot or a vaginal orgasm. The advantage is that you're already fully aroused. Your clitoris has already swollen to its full size and is extra sensitive thanks to climax number one, which maximizes the chance of you finally scoring another orgasm.

DON'T COMPARE YOURSELF

What works for friend A or friend B may not necessarily work for you, too. Everyone's bodies are different and have other user instructions. Practice and experiment a lot (solo and with a plus one) to discover the magic combinations for you.

The Art
of Coming

Four people who know a lot about sex share their secrets

Barbara Carrellas *is the founder of Urban Tantra, an approach to conscious sexuality that adapts and blends a wide variety of sacred sexuality practices from Tantra to BDSM. She is the author of* Urban Tantra: Sacred Sex for the Twenty-First Century—*now in its second edition*—Ecstasy is Necessary: A Practical Guide to Sex, Relationships and Oh So Much More, *and* Luxurious Loving. *Her books, workshops, and lectures are an eclectic mix of sexual and spiritual practices designed to encourage readers and participants of all genders and sexual preferences to expand their capacity for both pleasure and spiritual fulfillment. You can find her on Twitter and Instagram (@urbantantrika) as well as on Facebook, and read more about her and her work at barbaracarellas.com.*

66 The secret to a long, deep, magic-carpet-ride of an orgasm is something you're already doing regularly—you're breathing. All you have to do is breathe a bit more fully and deeply than you usually do, and—here's the tricky part—keep breathing all the way up to and into your orgasm. No holding your breath! For most of us (including me) holding our breath as we approach orgasm is the number-one habit to break in order to step into the universe of long, deep orgasms. So, practice, practice, practice. This practice is best done by yourself so you can really focus on your breath. You may find that the more you breathe the 'farther away' your orgasm feels. It may even feel like all the breathing is shoving your orgasms away. Keep going! It will likely take you longer to reach orgasm, but when you do orgasm it will last a lot longer.

Think of it from an energetic fuel perspective. You want to have an orgasm so you raise sexual energy. When you've raised sufficient sexual energy, your orgasm 'takes off.' If you're not breathing much, you'll have only raised a teacup's worth of fuel and your orgasmic flight will be pleasant, but short. However, if you take your time and breathe a lot, you'll raise gallons and gallons of energetic fuel. When your orgasm takes off from that launching pad you can fly for a long, long time.

So, lie back, relax your jaw, open the back of your throat (a fake yawn will show you how to do this). Breathe in through your nose and exhale through your mouth. If you're not comfortable breathing in through your nose, feel free to breathe in and out through your mouth. The most important thing is to take in as much air as possible in a relaxed manner. Now masturbate. Keep breathing! More breathing! Still more breathing!

Enjoy your orgasmic flight. **"**

Lorrae Jo Bradbury *is a sex, love, and empowerment coach whose sex-positive work helps the erotically curious to overcome shame and navigate kink, poly, and queer identities. After founding* Slutty Girl Problems *in 2011 to destigmatize sexuality and reclaim "slut" as an empowering term, she now focuses her efforts on supporting others with tools for deep self-love, sensual embodiment, and authentic communication. You can find her on Instagram (@lorraejo) and read more about her and her work at lorraejo.com.*

" One of my favorite ways to experience orgasm is through something not many people have heard of . . . sex magic! A practice wherein I harness the power of my pleasure to help me reach my goals and create a life aligned with all that I desire. It truly has transformed my life, literally training my brain to associate my goals with erotic pleasure until simply thinking about them can begin to elicit that orgasmic sensation. When I first started practicing sex magic, it was incredible: The results were noticeable almost immediately. I couldn't wait to start working on new projects and was overflowing with motivated energy, even at times when I was feeling tired and run down!

It might sound impossible, but it's actually pretty easy—and you can start any time. You don't need a partner to do it. In fact, it's actually more powerful to perform it solo when you're just starting out.

There are a lot of different ways to practice sex magic, but I like to keep it simple. What to do: Instead of thinking about erotic fantasies while you masturbate, think about your goals in vivid detail. Envision every nuance of what your life would look like, focusing especially on how reaching that goal would make you feel. Allow this vision to be the fuel for your orgasmic pleasure.

As a beginner's tip, you can start with your usual fantasies—erotica, a tantalizing film—then as you approach the peak of pleasure and orgasmic inevitability, switch to visualizing your goal-oriented desires. Even just a few moments of connecting pleasure to your goals can have an incredible impact.

This practice has helped me to envision the future that I want to create for myself in vivid detail, and created a kind of Pavlovian pleasure response towards my goals. I now associate my ideal vision of the future with so much pleasure that I'm extremely motivated, inspired, and energized to work toward it in my everyday life. In this way, sex magic has brought more sensual pleasure into every aspect of my life and experience—not just during sex! It's the kind of an orgasm that can literally change your life. 🍯🍯

Dorian Solot *is a sex educator and co-founder and director of Sex Discussed Here!, which for more than a decade has provided smart, funny sex education programs at colleges, conferences, high schools, churches, and many other venues across the United States. She is the coauthor of* I Love Female Orgasm: An Extraordinary Orgasm Guide *and has been featured on numerous programs and networks and in numerous publications from* The Early Show, CNN *and* NBC *to* The New York Times, NPR, The New Yorker, *and more. You can learn more about her and her work at ilovefemaleorgasm.com.*

❝ The Magic of Ten game is a fun way to expand your orgasm repertoire and learn to have more intense orgasms. Start in your favorite orgasm position and masturbate almost to the brink of orgasm, but stop before you reach 'the point of no return.' That's one.

Change positions: If you were lying on your back, try kneeling, or sitting with your back against the wall. You'll lose some arousal, but not all. Start touching yourself again. It might be a bit more challenging this time, because you're not as accustomed to doing so in this position. Once again, stop before letting yourself have an orgasm. That's two.

Repeat, changing positions each time—this will take some creativity! Experiment with lying on your side, crouching doggie-style, or putting your legs closer together or farther apart than you usually do.

When you reach ten, allow yourself to enjoy falling over the orgasmic edge, with the heightened sensations that typically come with a longer buildup. It can be liberating to realize your body has the potential to come in so many different positions. And if the game doesn't go as expected, that's fine, too—make up the rules as you go along. There's no way to lose at a game that ends in orgasm! **"**

Marla Renee Stewart, MA, *is a sexologist, sex coach, and owner and founder of the sexuality education company Velvet Lips, as well as a cofounder of the Sex Down South Conference. With more than twenty years of experience studying human sexuality, she has conducted over four hundred workshops all over the world and has been featured on a variety of media outlets, including Netflix's* Trigger Warning with Killer Mike *and* Love & Hip Hop: Atlanta. *Along with Dr. Jessica O'Reilly, she is also coauthor of* The Ultimate Guide to Seduction & Foreplay: Techniques and Strategies for Mind-Blowing Sex. *You can stay up to speed on her and her work at velvetlipssexed.com and on Instagram and Twitter,* @1marlastewart.

"It can't be said enough: Hands down, the best way to achieve mind-blowing orgasms is through erotic breath work and conscious breathing. Inhaling through your nose, breathing deeply down into your genitals, and exhaling through your mouth can lead you to some really powerful orgasms. By concentrating on your breath, you're able to stay focused, present, and centered on yourself and your pleasure so that you're fully experiencing every sensation. Through this simple technique, you can find different points of sexual awareness in your body, which can be extremely beneficial for you and your lover(s)—and when you combine this deep breathing with pelvic contractions, that's even more the case!

If you're not a generally anxious person, try flexing your pelvic floor muscles and squeezing while there is clitoral or vaginal stimulation for a more grounding experience. (If you do tend to be more anxious, you can nix the pelvic floor exercises and just concentrate on steady breathing that leads from shallow breathing in the neck to deeper breathing in the stomach and then finally down to the genitals.) Combining the breath work with the pelvic floor movement can create an intense euphoric experience, and if you breathe, relax, and let the energy flow, you'll likely ejaculate! It's as simple as that. There are so many benefits that come from simply breathing consciously and centering your mind, breath, and movements completely on your pleasure. 🙴

3

Orgasm, orgasmore, orgasmost

How to graduate cum laude in coming: eight techniques for reaching higher peaks

Issa: Trying to fuck is hard.
Molly: No it's not. It's like riding a bike.
Issa: Yeah, I don't know how to do that either.

Issa Dee and Molly Carter in *Insecure*

Lengthy foreplay

There are three major misconceptions about "foreplay": 1) Foreplay consists of "manual work" and oral sex only; 2) Foreplay might as well be skipped; 3) You can only have an orgasm after foreplay and penetration.

1. Foreplay consists of "manual work" and oral sex only

"Foreplay" is best defined as warming up for a bout of sex (which is not by definition penetrative sex, as we've already discussed on page 14). And that could be anything—you get to decide. That's the beauty of it. From sexting to watching porn together, from a foot massage to anilingus: Whatever floats your boat . . .

2. Foreplay might as well be skipped

It doesn't take much for an AMAB penis owner's body to be ready for sex. An erection and they're raring to go (although that's not a foregone conclusion for every person). A vagina owner's body, on the other hand, needs time to prepare for penetration. As you now know, on average it takes you twenty minutes to become fully aroused. That time is needed for the production of fluid and the creation of space. Are you jumping the gun? In that case, sex can be painful. If you don't self-lubricate easily, you can use a bit of lube, but don't see this as a substitute for foreplay. When the lube dries up, you'll start chafing inside. And that's not much fun.

Then again, not everyone needs a full half hour to get limbered up. Some get wet faster than others. It's important to know this about yourself, so you can tell an impatient bed partner that they can't enter or put anything inside you just yet. Foreplay is recommended for maximizing your sexual arousal and boosting your chances of an orgasm, but it offers no guarantee. There are many other relevant factors, like attraction, techniques, and your frame of mind.

3. You can only have an orgasm after foreplay and penetration

"Foreplay," penetration, orgasm, and perhaps a bit of "afterplay." We're often taught that this is the right order of having sex. News flash: There is no "fixed order" for sex. That said, we do recommend some form of foreplay for pain-free and pleasurable penetrative sex. So what if the two of you come during foreplay and then both roll over and catch some Zs? Fine! "Sex" is often associated with penetration, but that's usually the moment for a penis owner to shine. Vaginal penetration does relatively little for the vagina owner's orgasm, unlike cunnilingus and fingering. What many define as "foreplay" (a hand job, fingering, a blowjob, or cunnilingus) can be the entrée and not just the appetizer. Oral sex is sex, too. A hand job is sex, too.

Fifteen foreplay ideas

Trying out new things is the secret to an unpredictable and (more) exciting sex life. Think outside the box and beat the routine. You'll go far with these fifteen playful tips.

SEX GRAB BAG

Together with your lover write down all kinds of ideas about sex positions, locations, role play . . . you name it. Put the pieces of paper into a jar without telling each other what you wrote. Agree to pull a note out of the "grab bag" and act on it every once in a while. The anticipation is part of the fun!

ROLE PLAY

When you've been together for a while and you know each mole and stray hair inside and out, your sex life will benefit hugely if you occasionally step out of your comfort zone. Role play will introduce you to a whole new side of yourself and your lover. Fulfill long-cherished sexual fantasies. Classics like the nun, student, and attractive stranger are a few popular hits. And the Oscar goes to . . .

THE FOOD OF LOVE

What's that saying, the way to love is through the stomach? So is the way to lust! Arrange traditional sex foods on the bed—ice cream, chocolate, strawberries, whipped cream, cherries, and cake come to mind. Take time feeding each other all these delicacies, sucking on each other's fingers, and licking the cream off each other's body. And don't worry about making a mess. Round two can start with a shower.

KEEP YOUR UNDIES ON
Feeling a boner or finger on your clit with only a thin piece of fabric in between—do you remember the exhilaration of "dry humping"? That thrill of almost, but not *quite* naked is a huge turn-on. Sometimes you feel more exposed wearing a single item of clothing than nothing. Keep your undies on during "foreplay" and let your partner have a sneaky feel inside your panties. Arousal assured.

MISSING PANTIES
On a date? Slip to the bathroom mid-evening and take off your panties. Return to the table and drop the piece of fabric into their lap. You'll be skipping dessert!

THRILLING
While out and about, take a vibrating toy you can wear inside your vagina and hand the remote to your partner. You'll be heading home with screaming tires!

GOING PLACES
Going to a dinner, birthday party, the movies, or a wedding? Be a tease and hitch up your skirt or dress (or if you're more into pants—pick some convenient times to bend over) from time to

time. You can bet your partner won't be able to keep their hands off you all night.

PLAYING IN THE PARK
Feed each other fruit in a sun-drenched park or in the garden. Back off whenever they try to kiss you and turn it into a game. If you want to risk it, you can indulge in a bit of alfresco sex (so long as you're in a completely private area—there are laws, after all!).

TRAIL OF CRUMBS
Is your partner home late? Throw a surprise party. . . . Leave a trail of clothing from the front door to your sex location where you welcome them in a sexy pose.

READING
Surprise your lover by reading them an erotic story about your ultimate fantasy. Adopt your sultriest voice (Scarlet Johansson, maybe, as an inspiration?) and gradually remove your clothes.

GETTING STEAMY
You can have "foreplay" wherever you like. Tired and "dirty" after a long day at work? Or fancy sex first thing, but you've got a case of the morning breath? Kill two birds with one stone by taking a shower together. Lather each other up and give a sexy massage. Start at the shoulders before slowly working your way down. Pay extra attention to the good bits. Go down on your knees and let your tongue do the talking.

STRIPTEASE

Who doesn't love a striptease? Why not go for it. Put on your favorite butt-shaking music and start peeling off your clothes. Too daunting? Practice in front of the mirror first and don't take it too seriously!

SPECIAL DELIVERY

A trench coat, sexy heels, and nothing else . . . or whatever your style's equivalent is! Then ring your partner's doorbell late at night. Surprise!

I SPY

When one sense is taken away, the others become keener. . . . Have yourself blindfolded and ask your partner to trace a feather all over your body. Linger at the erogenous zones: neck, throat, breasts, navel, and thighs. Let this flow into oral sex or a hand job. Like it a little kinkier? Then bring out the handcuffs or restraints.

WATCHING PORN TOGETHER

Choose a (ethical) porn clip that appeals to you both and re-enact the scene. That way you can try something new without having to improvise. The visuals will get you automatically aroused.

Breathing

Breathing. We all do it, but 90 percent of the time we're not truly aware of it. That's a shame, because breathing is an extremely powerful tool for controlling mind and body. It helps you to take your mind off things and it also leaves you wonderfully relaxed, which is essential for good sex. In chapter 2, you read that your breathing can help you to lift your peaks to an even higher level. Let's take a closer look.

Solo

Start by doing your breathing exercises in a neutral setting. Just you . . . in your loungewear with a cool instrumental track in the background. Then practice a couple of times while having solo sex. Once you've mastered this, you can show off your tricks to a plus one.

Go deep

Anyone who's ever done yoga will be at an advantage. You'll probably know that you need to breathe in through the nose and out through the mouth. Breathe in for seven seconds and out for eight. Make sure you breathe "deep and low," that is to say, from your abdomen. When you feel that your pelvic floor muscles are engaged, you're doing it right! You'll feel every touch and every tingling sensation so much more intensely. Tip: It helps to rest your hand on your lower abdomen.

Build-up

Slowly ramping up your breathing helps you to reach your peak faster. The closer you are to your climax, the faster you start breathing. Are you on the edge? Start breathing fast but deep. Remember to keep your body relaxed. Please note: Don't do this for too long, and skip it altogether if you're prone to hyperventilation.

Some people fare better when they breathe slowly and deeply. Try both approaches and see what works for you.

Synchronicity

Often, the stronger your bond with your bed partner, the better the sex. And the better the sex . . . exactly, the greater the chance of a climax.

Squeeze and release

The section about mental orgasm (see page 66) revealed that you can use your pelvic floor muscles to "think" yourself to a climax. You can use the same technique to come faster and more forcefully. By alternately squeezing and releasing your pelvic floor muscles, you stimulate the clitoris even more and bring your happy ending just that little bit closer. The nearer you are to your orgasm, the faster you go. Tip: Combine this with the breathing technique described above and achieving an orgasm becomes a cinch.

Warm versus cold

Hot or cold temperatures can provide the body's neuroreceptors with extra stimulation and send anybody into a state of ecstasy. Where warmth has a relaxing effect, cold produces endorphins, also known as happiness hormones. But remember: The penis and the cold are uneasy bedfellows. A clitoris, on the other hand, doesn't mind some cooling action, although it's not everybody's cup of tea.

Hot water
Here are some directions for your partner: Take a sip of hot water. Hold the water in your mouth for a while to warm things up in there. Then, swallow and place your warm tongue directly on the vulva. Let it rest there, to transfer the warmth. Then

swallow another sip of hot water, place your whole mouth over the labia, and lick the clitoris. Repeat this for as long as you like. But be careful, don't make it too hot. Scalded genitals are the ultimate mood killer.

Quickie

You can do the same thing to a penis owner! Take a sip of hot water, wait a moment, swallow, and spoil the balls and penis with your mouth. We're willing to bet that they won't hold out for very long.

Massage candle

You can also play with the heat of a candle. Light a massage candle and let it burn for about fifteen minutes. As an added bonus, it sets the mood and suffuses your home with a lovely scent. Blow out the candle and leave it to cool for a minute or so. Pour the wax directly onto the body or into your hands. Start off by massaging the back, buttocks, and legs. Take your time and don't miss any part of the body. Ask your partner to roll over and set to work on the front. Start with the mildly erogenous zones (throat, feet, navel) and then gradually move on to the breasts/chest and private parts.

Like it a bit naughtier? Use a blindfold to deprive your partner (or yourself) of vision. The other teases their blindfolded partner by slowly dripping candle wax over their whole body.

Please note: Only use candles that are especially made for adult bedroom activities to avoid burns. Regular candles tend to have a higher melting point. A massage candle is safe for all parts of the body, smells divine, and the wax doesn't harden.

Ice ice bae bae

It was a familiar trope in romantic films from the 1990s: Scenes featuring a couple slowly rubbing ice cubes all over each other's body. It's a cliché and for a good reason, as you can heat things up with something cold. Ask your partner to put an ice cube into their mouth and trace figures over your body . . . from your neck, down to your chest, past your navel, and to the inside of your thighs. Then your partner can lick the cold liquid off your skin again—in the same order. Ooh la la, you'll be getting all hot and steamy in no time!

Quickie
Safety first. Only use ice cubes made of water and stop playing if you feel a burning or itching sensation or your skin turns blue or bright red.

Glass dildos are made especially for safe cooling. Put the toy in the fridge for an hour before using it in the same way as the ice cube. If you like, you can then use it internally for an ice-cold sensation.

Stimulating creams

You can use stimulating substances to spice things up a bit. There are all kinds of creams, lubes, and condoms with a warming, tingling, or cooling effect. These aren't miracle drugs for a Big O, but a bit of experimentation can't do any harm.

Lights on versus lights out

"Women's" magazines are always urging us to do the horizontal mambo with the lights on because we shouldn't be insecure about our bodies. And sure, sex with the lights on enhances intimacy because you can look at each other (depending on your position, obviously) and receive sexy, visual input. But there's something to be said for sex in the dark . . .

Focus on you

Is your wandering mind getting in the way of a climax? Why not do it with the lights (almost all) out. It's easy to get distracted in a brightly lit room. In the dark, with your vision restricted, you're not only blind to the mess and your mental to-do list, but you'll automatically focus more on your body.

Let go

Insecurities about your skills and your body can give you a mental and physical "block" and make sex a struggle. Churning thoughts are an obstacle to pleasure and any chance of a Big O. If you need a dark room to feel comfortable during sex . . . then why the hell not? All at your own pace. But because you shouldn't worry about your performance or your body, we encourage you to introduce more light each time you have a tumble in the sack. Tip: Candles provide a beautiful, soft glow and create a sultry atmosphere at the same time.

Fantasy

Go on, it's safe to admit it. There are times when you fantasize about having someone else between your legs other than your partner. Don't worry, it's completely normal. According to a 2015 survey by the sex toy company Lovehoney, basically half of all women regularly fantasize about another partner or a different situation or activity during sex. And, you know what? The other half ought to try it! It's about fantasy, and for some this could be the necessary nudge toward orgasm. In the dark, it's a cinch to give free rein to your creativity. Hayley Kiyoko . . . Ryan Gosling . . . Indya Moore . . . is that you?

Edging

The greater the pressure, the brighter the diamond . . . right? The same goes for an orgasm. Edging is a technique in which you put off your happy ending for as long as possible. It results in an even more explosive orgasm. You can do it solo or with a partner, using a toy or fingers.

1. Stimulate your clitoris (or G-spot or whatever works for you) until you're about to come.

2. Stop the stimulation entirely and pause until the arousal has largely abated.

3. Resume the stimulation. . . .

4. Take another break when you're close to the edge.

5. Repeat this as often as you like before you fully surrender. . . . Curling toes assured!

Coming together

If mainstream Hollywood is to be believed, a climax happens through 1) penetrative sex and 2) simultaneously with a male partner. Um, not necessarily . . . but one thing is true: A joint trip to seventh heaven may be the most intimate experience there is. Luckily that's not a mission impossible. With the right steps you're bound to achieve it.

1. Practice

In order to come together, you'll have to become a pro at timing your orgasm. For this you need to know your body inside out. What moves do or don't work for you? Draw on this knowledge to either speed up or slow down your orgasm. Both of you need to figure this out solo before you get it on together.

2. Slow down or speed up

Successfully completed step 1? Discuss your findings, so you'll know what to do at the decisive moment. Compare how long, on average, it takes you to come and find the middle way. A possible method is for one to slow down and the other to speed up their orgasm. Getting a head start is a bit easier for both parties. Let yourself be pampered for fifteen minutes (or longer) before the other joins in.

Is your sex partner good at speeding up their orgasm? Use it to your advantage! Are you nearly over the edge and there's no return? Go ahead and holler. Your partner may be able to catch up so you can cross the finish line together.

> ### *Quickie*
> **The dual orgasm may be easier when your partner has already come once before. With the pressure off, they can keep going for longer.**

3. Multitask

In chapter 2, you read that the more zones you stimulate, the greater the chance of an orgasm. With only 10 to 20 percent of women reporting that they're capable of coming through penetrative sex alone, a finger or toy on the clit is essential for coming together. You can leave this to your partner, but because you've got a better idea of what you're feeling, it's easier to take matters into your own hands.

If you're after a synchronous climax during oral sex, the 69 is a gift from the universe. It may feel less romantic because you can't look each other in the eye, but that could also make it more exhilarating.

4. Communicate

The more often you sleep with someone, the better you're able to tell whether they are close to orgasm. That comes in handy when you want to finish simultaneously. But you need both verbal and nonverbal cues to communicate how far you are. Groan louder to indicate that you're getting closer, and use the simple, yet effective words "I'm coming" to let your partner know that they need to speed up.

5. Practice makes perfect

No luck at the first attempt? Don't worry, keep repeating the above steps and it'll come to you!

Babe, we need to talk . . .

How to turn sex into a hot topic (instead of a sore point)—and why no Big O is no big deal

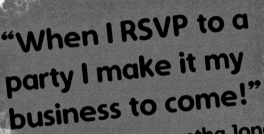

"When I RSVP to a party I make it my business to come!"

Samantha Jones in
Sex and the City

In order to close the orgasm gap—and, honestly? Just to have better sex!—we need to spring into action. Take charge. Call the shots. Seize control. Do you want an orgasm? Then you must (politely and consensually!) demand one, whether it's from your long-term relationship or a one-night stand. You're doing it for pleasure, right? But taking matters into your own hands is easier said than done. Sex is relatively easy. *Talking* about sex, however . . . is damn hard. It takes a bucket load of guts and self-confidence. There are three moments when you can issue directions to your bed partner: before, during, and after sex.

Why AMAB penis owners know what they want

One of the causes of the orgasm gap is that we tend to not explore our bodies enough. We're not familiar with our favorite moves and, in straight relationships especially, can tend to be eager to please our boo first. But AMAB penis owners kinda know their bodies inside out. They often know exactly how their joystick works and how they or someone else can best play with it. Why is that? From a young age, they see and feel their member daily. When they want sex, they get an erection. Because their genitals are on the outside, they automatically figure out how their body functions. But our genitals are mostly internal and therefore not as immediately visible. We also start masturbating later in life: Studies have found that by age 15, only 25 percent of young vagina owners have masturbated and reached orgasm compared to . . . nearly 100 percent of young AMAB penis owners.

Prior to sex

Be positive

Communicating about sex doesn't have to be awkward. Start doing it as early as possible in a relationship, so it becomes a habit. Make sure you also talk about what you enjoy. Saying things like "You never do this" or "you always do that" is an absolute no-go. Try beginning with a compliment before highlighting areas of improvement. Be honest, but sell it like constructive criticism.

Scared? Then say so

Are you nervous about broaching the issue? Then just say so. By showing your vulnerable side, you encourage your partner to be open-minded, understanding, and vulnerable, too.

Timing is everything

Carefully choose the moment and the location to talk about sex. Avoid blunt statements like, "Babe, we need to talk." Those words trigger stress. You might try to subtly slip the topic into the conversation, so things don't get too heavy—when you're watching TV, driving, or cooking together, or simply lying side by side in bed. That being said, open communication is a great thing in a relationship. If you and your partner are able to have open and honest conversations or are working toward it, don't be afraid to speak up!

No need for words

Can't get the words out? Here's a simple solution: Send a link to a video or an image of what looks hot to you, with the words, "Let's try this sometime." Another nonverbal trick is the sex grab bag from chapter 3. If you're afraid to say it out loud, write it down instead and put it in your lucky dip jar, whether it's role play, BDSM, or a particular type of orgasm.

Example phrases

I love it when you go down on me. It would be even better if . . .

I'd love it if we could come simultaneously.

I read about a different kind of orgasm. Let's try it.

I'd be really turned on if you did . . . to me.

During sex

Sometimes it's less awkward to issue pointers *during* hanky panky. You're already doing it anyway. Unlike pre-sex talks, it's essential that you be clear and concise. Talking in bed is essentially dirty talk . . . and you know how thrilling that can be. Talking dirty is an exciting and fun way to get what you want in bed.

**Also use words to express when there's
something you do NOT want. For instance,
when something's painful or your partner
doesn't respect your boundaries. And
remember it's always good to communicate
those boundaries beforehand, too!**

Plain speaking

A clearly structured argument with do's and don'ts about how to make you come is too much of a good thing. Short and sweet sentences work best. Don't just identify things that could be better, also indicate when you're enjoying yourself. That way they know that they're hitting the spot.

"Don't not have an orgasm. Make sure he knows that you're entitled to an orgasm. I like to say it. I'll be like: 'Hey, there are two people here.' I'll be like, 'Oh my God, have you met my clit?' Don't be self-conscious."

Amy Schumer in *Glamour*

Moan

Moaning is more than just a trick to facilitate a climax. You can use this form of nonverbal communication to indicate whether your partner is on the right track and whether you're getting closer to your happy ending. It's really simple. The closer you get, the louder you moan. Are they going off course? Lower the volume.

A helping hand

You don't always need words to give directions. Sometimes actions speak louder. Take hold of their hands or head (but be gentle) and steer them to the places that need attention.

EXAMPLE SENTENCES

Harder/gentler.

More pressure/less pressure.

Slower/Faster.

This is soo good.

Yes, right there.

A little higher/lower/to the left/to the right.

Massage my nipples.

After sex

"Evaluation" is unnecessary after a one-night stand, but if you're in a long-term relationship or plan on seeing the person again, it's good to exchange views during regular pillow talks. Be sure to emphasize the positive points and say—if applicable—what you'd like to see or do differently next time. And don't forget to ask what you can do better. It signals that they can be open, too.

EXAMPLE SENTENCES

That was awesome, next time I'd like to try . . .

What did you make of . . . ? How about I try . . . next time?

I'd find it super sexy if we do the position we just did in the shower next time while you play with . . .

You know the other thing I really like is when you use both your tongue and your fingers.

Showtime

Something that's both exciting and educational for your bed partner: showing them how it's done. Let them watch as you treat yourself on the bed (or wherever). Show exactly what you'd like them to do.

No big O, no big deal

Sex is like pizza—and the orgasm is the cheese. Without the cheese the pizza is perfectly palatable, but with it it's a whole lot tastier. Without a climax sex is less good, but not necessarily a fiasco. Not always having a blissful ending to sex? Many people can live with that. For others, it's a bigger problem. But one thing is certain: Sex can definitely be satisfying without a big bang at the end. . . . It all depends on how you do it.

Be in the moment
Performance pressure doesn't make it any better. Stress causes your mind and body to shut down. So don't just focus on the final destination, but enjoy the journey itself. And if you can't come, better luck next time!

Take your time
In a hurry to get to the finish line? Stop! Take your time. As long as there's attention to mutual pleasure, a bout of sex without *petite mort* can still be divine. Indulge in the sensual delights of oral sex and G-spot stimulation. Don't rush, but explore each other from head to toe. By incorporating the whole body, you build extra sexual tension. Even without experiencing a true peak, your body can tingle all over.

"Sex is always about emotions. Good sex is about free emotions; bad sex is about blocked emotions."

Deepak Chopra

Teamwork

Lovemaking doesn't always have to revolve around a climax. The physical and mental interaction between the two of you is center stage. Turn sex into something special from beginning to end. And that's highly personal to you. It can be a mutual erotic massage, candles and romantic music, and lots of eye contact. Or maybe thrilling power play, in which you assume the roles of a dominant and a submissive, is more your thing: Trust and surrender are at the core of BDSM. Coming is not the main purpose, but a nice byproduct.

Tantric sex

Tantric sex doesn't revolve around orgasm. On the contrary: Penetration itself often doesn't play any role at all. A connection with your bed partner lies at the heart of this eastern tradition. A tantric session can even last up to two hours! Want to have a go? You don't have to be a new age hippie to practice tantric sex.

OPEN-MINDED

For many, tantric sex is too "hippie-dippy" or outlandish. In practice, though, it's not that out there at all. The key thing is to be open-minded. Unless you open up to new things, you'll never experience them. So get rid of your prejudices and negative expectations and try to enjoy the moment.

IN THE MOOD

A relaxed pre-sex atmosphere is always good, but for tantric sex it's essential. Tantric sex largely depends on developing mental focus, so a nice ambiance is vital.

Create an atmosphere in which both of you feel relaxed. Take a steaming hot shower or a nice warm bath and pamper your body and each other with essential oils. Enhance the mood in the bedroom (or wherever you're doing it) with scented candles, ethereal music, and dimmed lighting. Make it cozy. Your safe spot. Take turns massaging each other with fragrant oil.

POSTURE

In tantric sex, the "positions" are just a little bit different from the norm. You either sit cross-legged facing each other or else you sit on your partner's lap with your legs wrapped around them.

LOOK AT EACH OTHER

Eye contact is an important element within tantric sex. Look each other straight in the eye. Do this for at least five minutes without saying a word. It may tickle your funny bone at first, but that's OK.

BE OPEN

Compliment each other while maintaining eye contact. Say what you think is cute, fun, or beautiful about the other person. Both inside and out. Take turns doing this and listen carefully to what the other is saying.

Follow this by sharing your sexual desires. What do you enjoy? What do you need? What would you like to try? Focus mainly on the mental and less on the physical aspect.

BREATHE TOGETHER

Enhance your connection even further by synchronizing your breathing. Take deep and slow breaths in and out and gradually establish a pleasant breathing rhythm. Breathing together and maintaining eye contact allows you to tune into each other even more and momentarily feel alone in the world together.

TANTRIC MASSAGE

From the eye contact and breathing exercises you can move on to a massage. Take your time, because we can't stress this enough: Tantric sex doesn't revolve around the orgasm, but around the connection. Now's the time to apply a sensual massage oil (if you haven't already). Caress your lover's body all over with attention. Use slow and firm strokes, up and down and from left to right. And the other way around. Include the erogenous zones, but also keep massaging the entire body. Do this long enough and they will grow completely relaxed and perhaps experience an all-over tingling sensation. It's up to you both whether you want to keep going and seal the deal . . .

5

Orgasm problems

What to do when you're not coming

"Fuck me badly once, shame on you. Fuck me badly twice, shame on me."

Samantha Jones in *Sex and the City*

While it's no big deal if you occasionally miss out on an orgasm, you often do long for that cherry on the cake, the cheese on the pizza, or the ketchup with your fries. That's why this chapter is a one-stop shop for all your orgasm probs. Think of it as the troubleshooting part of this guide—with reminders, tips, tricks, and advice on how to deal with the most common orgasm issues.

Difficulties coming

"Are you coming yet?" If we had a nickel for every time we heard this in bed . . . especially from our penis-owning companions—as if it's a race or some box you need to tick so you can move on to "the real work": their orgasm. Some people can come within five minutes, while others need up to ninety. In fact, it varies from one situation to the next, and even from one bed partner to another. Step one is to stop feeling ashamed of however long it takes for you. Every person is different and comes with a different user guide. It's not wrong to need more time. Don't let your sense of pleasure be overshadowed by this.

But it would be nice to have more control over your orgasm. It can be pretty frustrating when you're just not getting there. What to do? Step one: Find the cause.

Your partner

Let's be honest. Your inability to come could come down to your bed partner. It could be a question of poor "craftsmanship," or else your emotions may be interfering with your climax. Maybe you can't let yourself go because you don't have strong feelings for them. Start by building an emotional bond before you jump between the sheets. Are there any unsettled relationship issues that are getting in the way of your surrender and trust? It's said that you shouldn't go to sleep with an argument still on your mind. The same applies to having sex. Begin by talking through any underlying issues. Not only will you feel relieved, but you'll be able to open up again.

No instructions

Pointing the finger is oh so easy, but take a look at yourself, too. Are you standing up for your right to a climax? Are you giving your bed partner enough guidance? Or are you leaving them to their own devices? Issuing direct instructions can feel awkward at first, but after a while it starts to feel normal. Return to chapter 4 for more on how to approach this, if you need.

"It's just that all men are sure it never happened to them and all women at one time or other have done it, so you do the math."

Sally, on fake orgasms, in *When Harry Met Sally*

Faking it

The worst thing you can do for your own pleasure is faking an orgasm. Sure, you're avoiding an awkward conversation and you're not hurting the other person's feelings. But . . . you're also doing yourself a disservice. Your partner will think they've done something good and will repeat those moves . . . and that makes it trickier to discuss things later on. The vicious circle continues . . .

Mindset

Is your head 100 percent in the right place? You become your own worst enemy when your negative thoughts get the upper hand. As soon as you think, "I won't be able to do it," you've given up in advance. But being too focused on your orgasm won't help either. If you are, the stress dominates and stops you from relaxing. And that's the biggest orgasm killer.

Not aroused enough

Without arousal your clitoris won't be fully engorged and without a fully engorged clitoris it's impossible—or certainly much less easy—to achieve an orgasm. So take plenty of time to warm up. Have another look at chapter 3.

Not coming with a partner

"A bit to the left. No, too far. Whoa, not too hard. Hey, my clit's not a turntable!" Do you recognize these thoughts? Many people can only dream of having an orgasm during sex with a partner. It's a particular issue for straight women: As we've said before, just 65 percent always come during sex, compared to 95 percent of men. But while a lot of penis owners are often not sufficiently familiar with a vagina owner's body, we have to take responsibility for our own pleasure, too.

There are many different reasons for not being able to come with a partner. . . . Do you know your own body well enough? Do you feel an emotional (or physical) bond with the other person? Is your head in the right place? Does the sex have all the ingredients you crave? Are you indicating what you want? If your answer to any of these questions is "no" then you can work on those things. But please note: Physical impairments and illness can play a role, too. More on this later.

Go on a solo mission

As we've mentioned already, AMAB penis owners experiment with their genitals from an early age. Vagina owners are often late bloomers in this area. Usually, it's not until we really get started with sex (in whichever way) that we start diddling in our undies. But even then, some of us continue to depend on our bed partners. We give them the reins and allow ourselves to be led. We need to find a better balance.

Communicate

We can't stress this enough. Communication is key. Another person can't look inside your head and feel what you're feeling. That means that you need to give instructions. Before, during, or after sex. Start doing this early on in your relationship, so that you both become used to it. Don't say, "You're doing it all wrong," but, "I love it when you do this or that." Be honest and be prepared to listen, too: What can you do better in bed? In chapter 4 you can read more about communicating about sex.

Words aren't effective? Then it's a case of show don't tell. Some people (men especially) learn better from visual cues. Place a hand between your labia and place their hand on top. Masturbate in your usual way. This enables them to familiarize themselves with the rhythms you like. Do this again later, but this time let them watch so they can see what you're doing with your fingers. Keep practicing and they'll know all the tricks of the trade in no time.

Be inventive

Many roads lead to Rome. You can come in lots of different ways. According to one study, only a quarter of women can come through penetration by a penis or a sex toy alone. If you can, then great, but if you're not one of those people, let it go. Let your partner stimulate your clitoris, do it yourself, or use a sex toy.

"No woman gets an orgasm from shining the kitchen floor."

Betty Friedan

Be confident

Communicating what you like is essential. But don't get fixated on one particular way. Does your partner do things just a little bit differently than you? Don't be frustrated—it will never be exactly the same as during your solo sessions. And that's just as well, since an orgasm with a partner often feels different anyway. Most people experience a more intense and longer climax.

Keep practicing

Rome wasn't built in a day, to add another Rome-related saying into the mix. First-time sex with somebody is hardly ever the best. You need to learn how best to respond to each other. But even if you've been together for years, it's never too late to work on your sex life! Keep working towards your orgasm, communicating during sex, as well as trying new things. Think of a new location, different positions, or try a new toy. Novelty = increased arousal = more blood to the clitoris = greater chance of an orgasm.

Not being able to come alone

You can get an orgasm with a plus one, but not solo? That's rough, because ideally we'd rather not be dependent on another person to send us over the moon. There are all kinds of reasons why solo sex may not culminate in a happy ending.

Don't feel guilty
The idea that masturbation is wrong and coming is allowed only with a (regular) partner are hopelessly outdated of course. But because masturbation remains a bit of a taboo subject, these feelings can still haunt you. Some people feel guilty during or after masturbation. This doesn't do much for your arousal and stops you from fully surrendering to an orgasm. So remember: Why feel bad about something that feels so good? Masturbation without guilt is the ultimate form of self-love.

Stimulate your senses
Masturbation and sex with a partner are quite distinct. We may have all kinds of reasons for "flicking the bean"; we don't always do it out of sheer horniness. Sometimes we service ourselves in order to sleep better or just to relax. Like the reason, the experience itself is totally different, too. During a solo session you miss the sexual stimuli of another naked and warm body above or below you. And that may be just what you need to get yourself over

the edge. If that's the case, you can boost your pleasure during masturbation to another level with visual stimulation. Yes, we're talking about porn! Ethical porn, to be precise. Scent plays a role, too. The smell of your familiar bed partner may make you feel comfortable and relaxed. That feeling can be the decisive factor for your Big O. So take good care of your nose during me-time. Shower with a nice gel and light some scented candles or incense before you jump between clean, crisp sheets.

Take the time to experiment

An orgasm is impossible without both physical and mental arousal. You need the perfect combination of stimuli to climax. If only a partner can bring you to a climax you may be missing a certain level of dexterity. How often and how long do you experiment with yourself? Embark on a solo voyage of discovery to the mental and physical elements that light you up . . . and those that don't. These could be dissimilar from your preferences with a partner. That's why an orgasm with a "helping hand" feels very different from a solo orgasm. No better or worse—just different. Again, it varies from person to person. Try a range of scenarios and learn what works for you.

Not being able to come—period

According to some studies, half of all women regularly struggle to achieve a Big O. In fact, some have such persistent orgasm problems that they've never achieved one. Or they used to get there, but then suddenly couldn't anymore (possibly due to specific circumstances). This is known as anorgasmia. An estimated 10 to 15 percent of women grapple with this.

"There is unbelievable power in ownership, and women should own their sexuality. There is a double standard when it comes to sexuality that still persists. Men are free and women are not. That is crazy. The old lessons of submissiveness and fragility made us victims. Women are so much more than that. You can be a businesswoman, a mother, an artist, and a feminist—whatever you want to be—and still be a sexual being. It's not mutually exclusive."

Beyoncé in *Out* magazine

Culprits

In 90 percent of cases anorgasmia has a psychological cause. For 5 percent of people, the cause is physical. A lack of (good) sex education and taboos surrounding sex can play a role, too. Here's a list of some of the reasons:

- Sexual trauma like rape or assault
- Pelvic floor disorders
- Stress or burnout
- (Chronic) illness
- Medication like antidepressants and contraceptives
- Fear or shame triggered by a taboo, religion, or insecurity
- Lack of sex education
- Fear of pain or of sex in general
- Feelings of guilt, perhaps over cheating
- Problems in your relationship
- Insecurity about sexual orientation
- Disinterest due to negative experiences
- Hormonal imbalance because of pregnancy, breastfeeding, contraception
- Drug and/or alcohol abuse

> **❝** I've always had difficulties coming. Masturbation felt weird, like I wasn't allowed to touch myself. 'Am I meant to feel like this?' 'Am I doing it right or is it me?' All kinds of negative thoughts would be swirling around in my head. When I started experimenting with boys, coming remained a big mystery. My insecurity only grew. I tried everything. Fingering, oral sex, different techniques, watching porn. . . . Nothing helped. But then I entered into a long-term relationship and began to have sex on a regular basis. Suddenly I had this feeling I'd never had before! Finally, an ORGASM! My first solo climax came when I tried the Zumio vibrator. For now, I only get orgasms during sex and when using the toy. It depends on the position, but I find the cowgirl particularly effective. I've never come through oral sex or fingering. Hopefully I'll manage it one day. **❞**
>
> *Jane (24)*

What to do

Anorgasmia isn't a life sentence. It can often be treated. How? The right method depends on the underlying cause. If it's sexual trauma, you'll need professional help. But if it's fear, lack of know-how, or guilt, you can work on it yourself.

DISCOVER YOUR SEXUAL SELF

Were you raised with the idea that sex is dirty, only for married couples, and that masturbation is dirty and wrong? These deep-rooted beliefs may be blocking your orgasm. Have a word with those little voices. Besides, maybe you're not familiar with your own sweet spots—you don't know whether you're close to a climax, or you're unable to give your bed partner(s) the right instructions. Lock yourself into the bedroom one rainy Sunday for a little me-time. Discover which mental and physical stimuli light your sexual fire. You can then pass this info on to your sex partner(s). Try new things, alone and with a sex buddy. You'll be rewarded with more excitement and more arousal. And, who knows, maybe to a climax!

MAKE DEMANDS

Whether you've been married for thirty years or you're having a one-night stand . . . tell the other person what you want. Some people tend to be pleasers; they lie back and wait to see what's coming to them (no pun intended). Nice as that may be, don't just wait your turn. Speak up! The other person can't see inside your head. Demand lengthy foreplay with attention to the erogenous zones that turn you on the most. "Kiss my neck," "Squeeze my nipples," "Use your tongue/fingers"—that kind of thing.

Say all this in your sultriest voice and success is assured.

Flip back to chapter 4 for more tips on sex talk.

FOREPLAY IS YOUR BEST FRIEND

In many cases, we can't come because our partners lack the necessary technical expertise. Change the focus of the sex to maximize arousal. Take all the time you need, half an hour if you have to! And instead of following your usual routine, try new techniques, positions, and rhythms, and explore all of your body's erogenous zones. Remember: Don't descend on that clit right away. Foreplay can be something semi-nonsexual like a massage. You need this relaxed, slow build-up—especially when coming is difficult—so that your clitoris and the walls of your vagina are fully engorged and sensitive.

Have another look at chapter 3 for tips on the various tricks and techniques to facilitate an orgasm.

TALK ABOUT IT

A lot of people can talk for hours with their friends about love and sex. But not necessarily when there's little happening in bed. Erectile dysfunction or not being able to come—we're not quick to volunteer such serious subjects. That's why it often feels like you're the only one grappling with a problem. Nothing could be further from the truth. Nobody experiences fireworks in the bedroom every single time. That's why opening up about your negative experiences is such a good thing. It will prompt others to share candid revelations, too. Who knows, perhaps someone else is going through something similar so you can level with each other. Or somebody managed to come out the other end and offer you some great advice.

But don't just talk about it with your friends, discuss it with your main squeeze, too. They can join you on a voyage of discovery to find out what does or doesn't work for you. Make it a habit to talk about your sexuality and you'll soon become better attuned to each other.

BRING IN THE BIG GUNS

Some people like gentle and indirect stimulation of the clitoris, while others thrive on vigorous rubbing. Are you in the second group, but just can't get over the edge? Who knows, perhaps a powerful vibrator will offer a solution. Chapter 7 looks at sex toys.

SEEK PROFESSIONAL HELP

When anorgasmia or the absence of sexual pleasure is the result of, for instance, sexual abuse, heavy medication, or illness, lengthy foreplay or a sex toy won't be enough. To (once again) enjoy sex and have an orgasm, you'll need to turn to a professional. This is also a wise move when the guilt or the taboo are so deep-seated that you can't work things out on your own or with someone else (if you're in a relationship). Explain your problem to your family doctor. They will recommend—depending on your situation—whether you're best off with a gynecologist, sexologist, or psychologist.

"I demand that I climax. I think women should demand that. I have a friend who's never had an orgasm in her life. In her life! That hurts my heart. It's cuckoo to me. We always have orgasm interventions where we, like, show her how to do stuff. We'll straddle each other, saying: 'You gotta get on him like that and do it like this.' She says she's a pleaser. I'm a pleaser, but it's fifty-fifty."

Nicki Minaj in *Cosmopolitan*

Dryness: not getting wet

When your body and mind receive erotic stimulation, the land down under wakes up. Blood flows to your labia, vagina, and clitoris. Your labia swell and turn a darker red, your vagina becomes wider and more elastic, your cervix "withdraws," and your clitoris swells.

Lubrication is an extremely important condition for sex (be it oral or manual or penetrative). Glands in your inner labia and inside your vagina produce fluid that facilitates sliding in and out of your vagina and over your clitoris. In a word: You become wet. Just how wet varies from person to person. Desert conditions can make you feel really insecure. That's unnecessary of course. There are several explanations.

Not enough foreplay

Lots of couples will resort to a generous dollop of lube or saliva to get the vagina wet, but this is not recommended. You ought to see these resources as a little "extra," not as a replacement. One of the causes of a dry vagina is insufficient arousal. If that's the case, your body isn't ready for sex . . . especially not for penetration. Even rubbing the clitoris can be painful. Key elements for foreplay are the right atmosphere and mindset, relaxation, breathing, and taking your time. Have another look at chapter 3.

Hormonal changes

As a vagina owner, you're probably all too aware that hormones aren't always your best friend. Most of us are familiar with mood swings, zits, and cravings. Medications like the contraceptive pill, antidepressants, antihistamines, and of course hormone therapy can affect your hormonal balance. If you go through menopause, your body produces less estrogen and progesterone, resulting in thinner and drier vaginal walls. The same is true when breastfeeding. The breastfeeding hormone lowers estrogen levels, which can in turn lead to vaginal dryness.

Vaginal care

Your vagina is a self-cleaning organ. How handy is that? But you do need to treat it well, or else things go wrong: Sex without a condom, washing with soap, or incorrect use of tampons and pads—your genitals don't like it. It disturbs their microbiome and leads to all kinds of discomfort—vaginal infections, bacterial vaginosis, and STIs—and can result in vaginal dryness, as does the use of special washes for your "intimate area," which is strongly discouraged by gynecologists. Rinsing your vulva and vagina with a bit of lukewarm water is enough. Your vagina will do the rest.

Use of condoms is a must if you want to prevent unwanted pregnancies and STIs. But there's another reason few people are aware of. When your partner dons a glove before you have sex, fewer bacteria will end up in your vagina. The same goes for an internal condom. Sperm can also upset the natural balance of your vajayjay (if your partner comes inside you), since it has a different pH value.

Likewise, tampons influence the microbiome inside the vagina. Wearing them too long can result in a desert between your legs. It's recommended never to wear a tampon longer than eight hours at a time. It's best to replace it every three to four hours, or even more regularly in the case of light flow. The material they're made of matters, too. Many tampon brands contain chemicals. Tampons made of 100 percent cotton can reduce vaginal symptoms like dryness, itching, and irritation.

Pregnancy, diabetes, and chemotherapy can likewise have a negative impact on vaginal wetness.

Are the symptoms not clearing up by themselves? Go and see your family doctor or a gynecologist.

Post-sex blues

The sex scored a solid 8 or higher, but as soon as you roll over a wave of sadness washes over you. You feel sad, irritable, anxious, and maybe even burst into tears. Sound familiar? You're dealing with a classic case of post-sex blues—or "postcoital dysphoria": an unexpected melancholic feeling that suddenly crops up after love-making. You're not the only one. In a study of around 230 college-aged women, 46 percent reported symptoms of postcoital dysphoria after sex—and other studies have shown similar results. Where does this feeling come from? Unfortunately, there hasn't been enough research to establish the exact cause. Sexperts think it's down to the generous dose of hormones produced inside the body when you come. So it's not that strange to experience such a big emotional release. "With everything that goes on in your brain during orgasm, it's hard to pinpoint one thing," according to sex researcher Debby Herbenick. "Your muscles have been tense and now they're relaxed, your heart rate was beating fast and now it's slower, your breathing was rapid and now it's gone down."

An occasional cry can't do any harm. Give your loved one a big hug and you'll feel right as rain again. But if it happens very frequently, it could be a sign of something else. Are you feeling happy and safe in your relationship with this person? Discuss it with them, a friend, or a therapist.

Headache during sex

As you read in chapter 1, an orgasm can be just as effective as a painkiller. In fact, some scientists claim that it's even better than popping a pill. A splitting headache? *Le petite mort* will alleviate the worst throbbing. But you can also get a headache during or after the deed. This is something that affects one in a hundred people. Some are hit every single time, whereas others experience it only occasionally. And people suffering from migraines are often familiar with sex headaches, too. Exactly when the pain occurs varies from person to person. Some start hurting during the arousal phase, others during orgasm or after sex.

The headaches can feel different, too. Pain during the arousal phase usually intensifies during sex. One variant is the throbbing, tension headache, which is sometimes accompanied by the sensation of a tight band around the head. A headache during the climax feels like a stabbing, severe pain that tends to ebb away again very fast. A post-orgasm headache is often throbbing and stabbing. The different types can alternate, too.

Calling a halt to a bout of sex because of a headache is a real pain but often necessary. Luckily there's a lot you can do.

An incipient headache while you're still getting turned on is often caused by muscle tension. Stop your foreplay and make sure you're in a comfortable position and not unnecessarily tightening your muscles. A relaxed and safe atmosphere is important to your physical and mental well-being. Take a hot bath or a warm shower to loosen up your muscles and to destress.

A stabbing pain during an orgasm is caused by changes to the blood flow in the brain. Unfortunately, there's not a lot you can do about this. If it's happening (more and more) often you should consult a physician. They can look for an underlying cause and, if necessary, prescribe medication. Also see your family doctor if the pain continues for a long time, is unbearable, or you're experiencing nausea, vomiting, or blurred vision.

Painful sex

According to the American College of Obstetricians and Gynecologists, about 75 percent of women generally have painful intercourse at some time. It's not surprising that your libido drops when you're experiencing little or no pleasure. Many people think pain is just a part of vaginal sex—that you have to "grit your teeth" before it gets better. That's so wrong. The abrasion can cause small tears inside the vagina, which in turn makes the next bout of sex unbearable. It can also lead to infections. Pain during one's first time having penetrative sex happens to a lot of people, but it shouldn't be a normal occurrence. Luckily it's a one-off for most.

Dyspareunia affects everyone, young and old. Some experience pain every now and then, others every single time. The causes, which are many, can be psychological as well as physical. These are the most common ones.

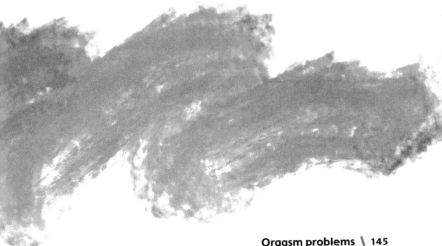

> **"One in ten women always experiences pain while making love: It seems fair to call that an epidemic."**
>
> **Ellen Laan, Dutch sexologist**

Not aroused

A dry vagina is the number one reason for pain during sex. And one of the causes of dryness is not being physically and/or mentally aroused enough. If you're not totally turned on, your clitoris isn't engorged, the entrance to your vagina isn't relaxed or wide enough, your cervix (if you have one) is still low, and your vagina hasn't produced enough mucosa (fluid).

Too tense

Fear and stress put the body—literally—on lockdown. Nothing can go in. Your pelvic floor muscles clench. An earlier experience of painful sex may mean that you "brace yourself." Everything below the belt screams: No way is anything coming in here!

STI

Genital warts, chlamydia, or a yeast infection can spoil the fun. These conditions make your vagina dry and penetration with a finger, penis, or toy painful. Look out for changes in and around your vagina. Can you see strange little lumps, is urinating painful, or do you have an itch? Take a peek at your underwear, too. . . . Has your discharge changed color or does it smell different? Seek help as soon as possible! If chlamydia goes untreated, it can leave some infertile. And an STI is nothing to be ashamed of. Visit a sexual health clinic or your family doctor and you can get back to making sweet, smooth love again in no time.

> ### *Quickie*
> **Never use soap to wash your vagina or vulva. Warm water is all you need. Soap upsets the natural acidity and increases the risk of a yeast infection.**

Hormonal imbalance

Your estrogen and progesterone levels can be imbalanced for a number of reasons, including the use of contraceptives. Those going through menopause may experience painful sex because their vagina is drier. During menopause, the body produces fewer hormones that normally lubricate the vaginal area. This can also affect those who are breastfeeding.

Endometriosis

In this condition, tissue similar to the lining of the womb grows outside the uterine cavity and attaches itself to your ovaries or fallopian tubes. It can also cause heavy and painful menstruation and bleeding between periods. The vagina loses flexibility, which can result in pain during sex. Do you have any of these symptoms? Don't suffer in silence. See your family doctor.

Vaginismus

When the vagina doesn't allow anything inside—no tampon, nothing—we're looking at vaginismus. The vagina is locked, so to speak. Penetrative sex is out of the question. This condition is not that easily cured. The underlying cause can be psychological or physical, such as a sexual trauma or overactive pelvic floor muscles after long and intensive exercise. Vaginismus can be treated through counselling from a sex therapist and through specific exercises.

What to do if sex is painful?

Below you'll find some general advice for help with painful sex. These suggestions are not specific to vaginismus, for which you should always consult a professional.

- Tell your bed partner immediately.

- Stop having sex and focus on pain-free activities that will enhance your arousal.

- Is penetration painful? Engage in longer "foreplay" (at least 30 minutes) so you're wetter.

- Take deep and slow breaths to help you relax.

- Don't use lube to solve the problem, but instead explore the issue!

- Consult a family doctor or sex therapist if the problem persists.

Assume your position

Orgasmic positions—straight or queer, partnered or solo

Missionary with pillows

WHY: There's nothing wrong with the good 'ol "missionary" position. It's a classic for a reason. But you can boost the pleasure level of this winner with some pillows. The higher your pelvis, the deeper your partner can go.

HOW: This is as easy as it gets. Place two or more (washable) pillows under your buttocks. Have your partner sit in front of you,

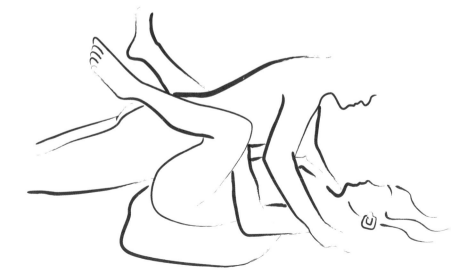

either on their knees or squatting. For stability—and for added force—they can hold on to your hips while thrusting. The higher the stack of pillows, the more pressure you'll feel on your clitoris. Ask them to press down on your lower belly (just above your pubic bone) with one hand and to massage your clitoris with the other. Hello, Big O!

VARIATION: This position also lends itself perfectly to a bit of muff-diving! With your buttocks raised, they have easy access to your vulva without having to twist their neck.

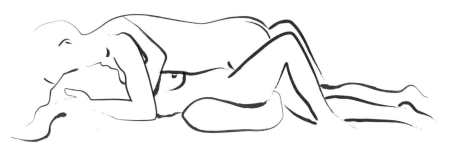

CAT

WHY: The Coital Alignment Technique is one of the few positions that's made for spoiling the glans of the clitoris. Many people who can come via penetrative sex do so via the CAT position. Try it and you'll find a whole new world open up to you.

HOW: This sex pose is similar to missionary, but the big difference is in the thrusting technique. Both of you are lying down, with your partner on top of you. Note that their chest is higher than yours. Place your legs at a 45-degree angle. Instead of moving up and down, they rock and grind or push against your pubic bone and draw circles with their hips. This creates maximum friction between their pubic bone and your clitoris. Oh, yes!

Reverse cowgirl (with a twist)

WHY: Do you like to be in control? Then welcome to your new favorite position. You're the one holding the reins in reverse cowgirl. You determine the rhythm, the tempo, and the depth. It's triple the fun for you because your G-spot is receiving stimulation—the

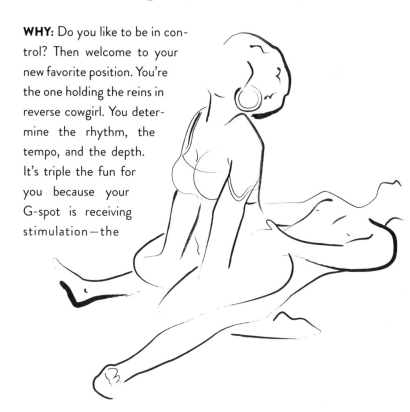

penis or dildo can move all the way in and out (the entrance to your vagina and the first two inches are the most sensitive!)—and you can pleasure your clitoris with your fingers or a sex toy. And let's not forget, your partner might love this position, too: They can lie back, with a great view of your rear—and, if your partner has them and you want to, you can pay attention to their *cojones*, too.

HOW: Your partner lies down with their legs slightly apart. You sit on top with your back to them. With your knees resting on the bed, you stick your legs under theirs. Hold on to their knees or upper legs for the necessary support. Slowly slide onto their member and move gently up and down. Gradually increase the tempo. It's up to you how deep you go. Alternate this with circling and rocking movements. Find a rhythm and a technique that you and your partner enjoy.

Use a vibrator or your fingers to stimulate your clitoris. Since you're in control of both penetration and clitoral stimulation, you can modify the rhythm, speed, and pressure needed for your Big O. If you time it well, you can come together!

VARIATION: Lean as far forward as possible for a different sensation for both of you. Or lean back a little for added pressure on your G-spot.

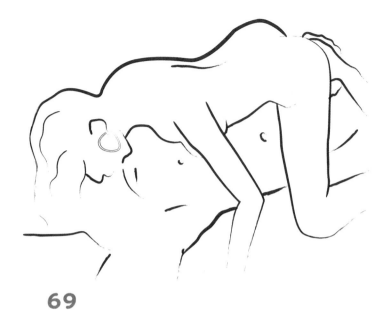

69

WHY: *Soixante-neuf* has a lousy reputation for some people. It's sometimes seen as a vulgar or filthy position, but as far as we're concerned, 69 doesn't get enough credit. It's more intimate than you think. You have lots of skin contact, you can give each other mutual pleasure, and—given enough practice—can come simultaneously. It's also a great position for anyone with sensitive breasts or nipples. Because they're dangling down when you're on top, more blood flows toward them and they become more sensitive. Gently rub your nipples across your partner's belly for extra stimuli.

HOW: The figures show it all. If your partner is a penis owner, you lie back to front so your mouth is close to their genitals. Conversely, their mouth can now reach your private parts. You're usually on top so you can decide how deep to take them into your mouth. If your partner is a vagina owner, place pillows underneath the buttocks and head of the person on the bottom. It makes it easier for you both to reach so you can lick and/or finger each other.

Voila! Now, give each other simultaneous oral pleasure. Be sure to pay attention to your partner's signals. The louder the moaning, the closer to orgasm. Are they getting there faster than you? Take a break, or switch to some gentler manual work. A drop of lube may also help them hold out a bit longer.

VARIATION: Move your hips from side to side or in circles, so they hit the best spots and you cross the finish line more easily. Sore neck? You can do *soixante-neuf* while lying on your side. Perfect for a lazy Sunday.

Quickie
Partnered with an AMAB penis owner? Keep an eye on the balls: They draw up closer to the body just before orgasm.

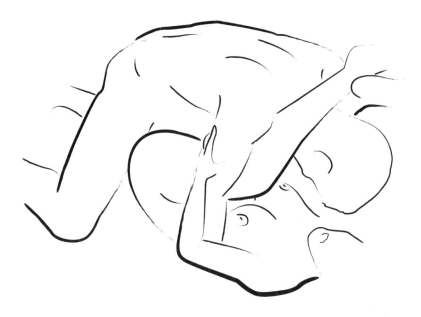

Viennese oyster

WHY: Deep, deeper, deepest! The Viennese oyster lends itself to exceptionally deep penetration. At this angle, the penis or dildo really presses up against your G-spot, and there's a lot of pressure on the (internal) clitoris. We guarantee you a truly dizzying sensation! Who knows, maybe it will give you an A-spot or P-spot orgasm. . . . Plus, this deep dive is extraordinarily pleasurable for penis owners, too!

HOW: As you can see, this position calls for some flexibility on your part. Lie down on your back with your legs in the air and have your partner sit in front of you. As they slide inside, they bend their upper body over you. Your legs move with them and end up somewhere around your neck. If you like, you can place a pillow underneath your buttocks for added intensity. You can also use a couples toy to come more easily.

But please note! This position can be too intense or painful for some people, so make sure that you're fully aroused and wet, relax your pelvic floor, and take deep breaths in and out.

VARIATION: Not a contortionist? Throw your legs over their shoulders and cross your ankles behind their head. Or ask them to hold your ankles and gently (!) push them as close as possible toward your head.

Doggy style

WHY: Doggy style feels very "primal" and therefore kind of exciting. It makes your partner feel alpha and you feel naughty. Not only are these roles a huge turn on for many, but your partner's tool can go really deep and provide maximum stimulation of your ultrasensitive G-spot.

People with sensitive breasts also like this position because their bosom receives additional stimulation from being flung from side to side. Tip: Lower your upper body far enough for your nipples to skim the mattress. The extra friction may be enough to push you over the edge.

HOW: Doggy style can be done in a variety of ways: both of you standing up, both on the bed, or with them standing and you on the bed. The principle is simple. They take you from behind while

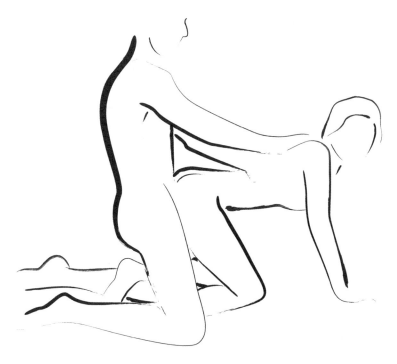

you rest on your hands and knees. Vary how far you push your knees apart. Close together gives an entirely different sensation than wide apart. Experiment and enjoy!

VARIATION: If you're not averse to a bit of butt play, you can ask them to gently massage your anus with their thumb.

> ## *Quickie*
> **Careful: "Doggy style" sex is not without risk.**
> **The position is known to cause the most penis**
> **fractures. Ouch!**

Lazy doggy

WHY: A fan of doggy style, but you'd like to up the pleasure and intimacy level? We present to you the lazy doggy. This position is more intimate, since you have more skin-on-skin contact. Plus, the pressure on your G-spot is even more intense thanks to the angle of your partner's thrusts.

HOW: In this position you're not on your four "legs," but flat on your stomach. Your partner lies flat on top of you. Spread your legs a little so they can lie between them. Or the other way around: You keep your legs together, while they place their legs outside yours—whichever you both prefer. Lift your behind so they can slide in more easily. Ask them to move horizontally for optimum G-spot stimulation. The higher you lift your butt, the deeper they can go. Oh. My. God.

TIP: Are they getting carried away? Lower your buttocks so they can't go as deep.

VARIATION: Try using a couples vibrator (see page 187) to reach orgasm.

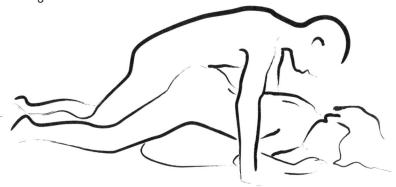

Lap dance

WHY: Are romance and connection high on your wish list? The lap dance is your go-to position. Although it can certainly enhance relaxation, nobody reaches a climax through romantic vibes alone. The lap dance is a delightful position if you like extra touching during sex. This position leaves your partner's hands free to caress, massage, and squeeze your upper body. Besides, you can also kiss on the mouth and the neck and suck each other's earlobes. The fact that you can see the pleasure on each other's faces only adds to the horniness.

HOW: Your partner sits cross-legged on the bed. You sit in their lap, facing them, and wrap your legs around their back. You take the lead: Move your hips back and forth and left to right. You can also move together, and with their hands on your hips you can find a rhythm that you both like. It takes a bit of practice, but once you're into the groove it's divine. To make it more intense, you can use a bullet vibrator or your partner can use their fingers to touch your clitoris.

VARIATION: Do you like penetration to be more intense? Let them grab your buttocks and move you up and down. Or put your feet on the floor so you can do it yourself.

Cozy cuddle

WHY: Intimate and exciting—these are the words for this cuddly position. It's just that little bit different, which gives the sex an edge. And you can boost your chances of an orgasm by playing with your nipples.

HOW: Ask your partner to sit up straight against the bedframe or the back of the couch. Sit in front with your back to them, so you're both facing forward. As they place both legs over yours you cross ankles (depending on how flexible the two of you are). With one hand they can massage your clit.

VARIATION: Turn your head for a sexy French kiss every now and then.

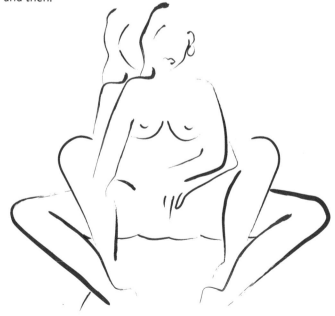

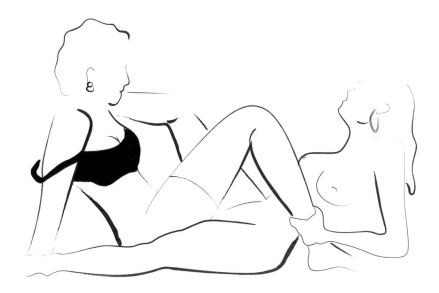

Scissoring

WHY: This one's for the queers! In this position, you can pay tribute to your partner's clitoris simultaneously and "hands free." It takes some practice, but eventually you may be able to climax together!

HOW: The position is called "scissoring" because it looks like two open scissors rubbing up against each other. It's a lot trickier than you think, because you need to be in exactly the right position. Make yourselves comfortable on your back. You both lift your right or left leg and place your foot either on the bed or over each other's shoulder. Make sure your clitorises touch before you start your gentle rocking and circular motions. Slowly increase the pressure, rhythm, and intensity. Give instructions and you're well on your way to coming together! If you like, you can place a vibrating toy between you for extra stimulation.

VARIATION: Instead of both of you having your buttocks on the bed, one of you can be the rider. Position yourself at right angles to each other's body and grind away.

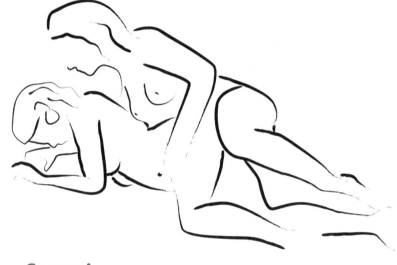

Spooning

WHY: Romantic, intimate, and ideal for those times when you don't want any "fuss." Simple and effective!

HOW: Ask your lover to lie on their side. Copy their position and lie down in front of them as the "little spoon." They can now reach your sweet spot with their hand. And not only that, but they can kiss your neck and suck your earlobe, too. Or maybe turn your head for a French kiss.

Double your pleasure by reaching back and massaging their clitoris, too. Is your arm too short? Bring in a wand vibrator.

VARIATION: Fancy even more pleasure? Ask your "big spoon" to use a dildo, vibrator, or strap-on. If your partner is a penis owner, they can enter you from this position, too.

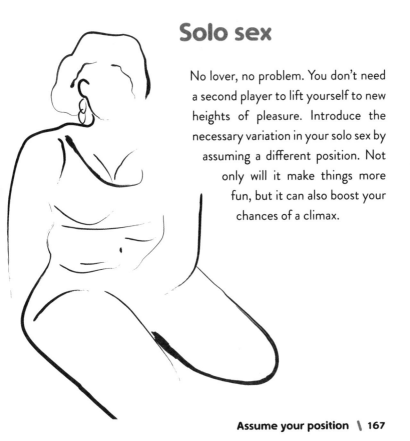

Solo sex

No lover, no problem. You don't need a second player to lift yourself to new heights of pleasure. Introduce the necessary variation in your solo sex by assuming a different position. Not only will it make things more fun, but it can also boost your chances of a climax.

Super star

WHY: Do you usually masturbate horizontally, that is to say, lying down? Experience a different sensation while going solo in a vertical position. Your blood will be flowing down faster, making your clitoris and vagina a lot more sensitive. It makes coming easier, and your peak much higher than normal.

HOW: Kneel down on a couch, chair, or bed with the top of your feet flat, so your legs are relaxed. Masturbate using your fingers or a sex toy, and don't miss sweet spots like your thighs and breasts or nipples.

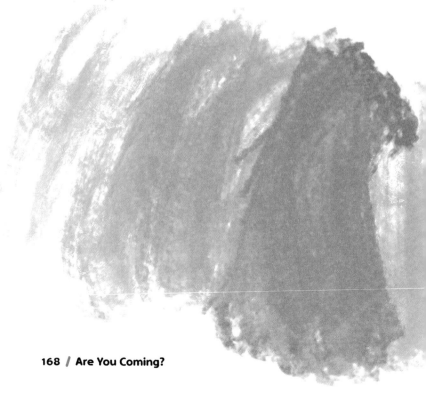

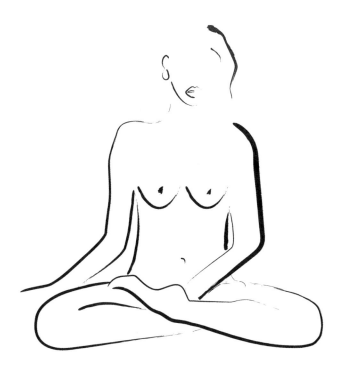

Lotus

WHY: Have you ever noticed how sexual yoga positions can be? The well-known lotus pose lends itself perfectly to a spot of diddling. With your private parts fully exposed, you can explore everything to your heart's content.

HOW: Sit cross-legged and place your left foot on your right knee. Do the same on the other side. Lean against a back rest or a wall for additional support. Let one hand (or a toy) do the work between your legs and use the other to explore your body. Some warm-up exercises and a yoga course are no luxury when doing this position. Not quite flexible enough yet? Just cross your legs—no need to put your feet on top of the knees. Keep practicing and you'll get there in the end!

VARIATION: Try this position lying on your back.

In the shower

WHY: As a teenager with raging hormones you may well have (accidentally?) discovered the magic power of the shower jet on your intimates. The average shower head is powerful enough to give you a climax. The fact that you're standing means you'll experience entirely different sensations than when you're sitting or lying down. Besides, the wet and warm setting of a bathroom is perfect for me-time.

HOW: Remove the shower head from its holder. Place your feet slightly apart and aim the water jet at your vulva. Move it in circles or up and down. If you like you can massage your breasts and nipples for extra stimulation.

Not everyone can come upright, because the sensation causes their knees to buckle. The solution is simple: Sit down. There's no risk of falling and it's more relaxing to boot.

VARIATION: If you feel up to it and are able to, you can select the showerhead's massage setting.

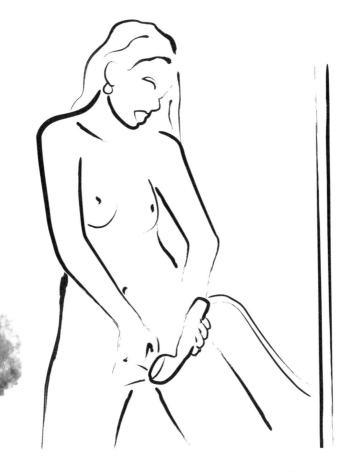

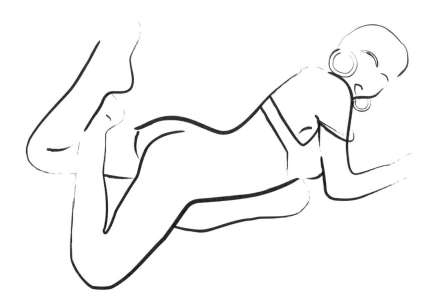

Flat on your stomach

WHY: Why not? Nine out of ten times, we lie on our back, so why not try to masturbate on your belly for a change. It feels a bit out of the ordinary.

HOW: Lie down on your stomach and put a pillow underneath your belly. Bend your knees and stick your butt up in the air. Slip your hand or a toy between your thighs. By tilting your pelvis and feeling more tension in your legs you'll make the experience more intense and a bit different.

VARIATION: Masturbate yourself with your other hand or (if you have long arms) via your butt instead of your belly.

The invisible man

WHY: No one at your disposal, but you fancy being on top? Use your imagination and simulate sex with the help of some toys.

HOW: Kneel down on your bed. Use a dildo or a thrusting vibrator (yes, they exist!) and a vibrator or air pressure stimulator to achieve a mixed orgasm: a climax through vaginal and clitoral stimulation. An explosion of bliss is guaranteed!

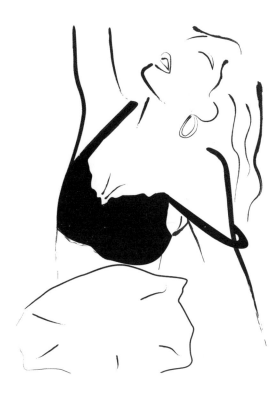

Couch surfing

WHY: Mix it up and have a solo session on the couch. The naughty idea that you're masturbating in a place where you might get caught is an extra turn on. Lying upside-down allows more blood to flow to your head and you may feel a little high.

HOW: Lie down on the couch and throw both legs over the back-rest (or lean them against the wall) and spread them wide enough for your knees to be outside your hip line. Let your head dangle over the edge of the seat. Use one hand for fingering and the other for playing with your breasts and/or nipples while holding on to the couch.

Remember, of course, to be careful! If you start to feel light-headed and think you should stop, move on to the next position.

VARIATION: This position also lends itself to oral sex. Ask your partner to kneel down in front of your face. They can then plea-sure you with a vibrator and/or knead your breasts.

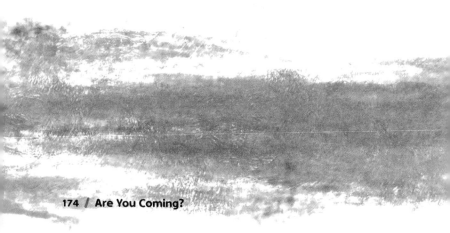

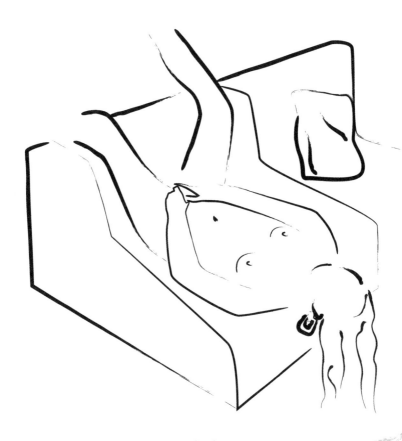

7

Let's play

Get the job done with sex toys

"Even if times are tough and you're enduring a terrible heartache, it's important to focus your anger on a vibrator, not another person."

Chelsea Handler

Toys, but for grownups. If you ask us, everyone ought to cram their bedside table full of vibrators, stimulators, couples toys, nipple clamps, and other exciting gadgets.

Which sex toys

There are hundreds of toys, but you may not have the time, money, or the inclination to try them all. Here we present the best that are worthy of a place in your bedside table.

Dildo
Vaginal, A-spot, and P-spot orgasm
Put simply: a fake dong. You can get them in all colors, with or without scrotum, veins, and suction cup—or even in useful shapes that don't look like a penis at all. The main difference with a vibrator is that a dildo does *not* vibrate. That's why it's a good replacement for penetration—you (or your partner) can move it up and down. Tip: During oral sex you can let the dildo rest inside your vagina for additional, mild stimulation.

Wand vibrator

Vaginal, A-spot, and P-spot orgasm

A wand vibrator is a perfect starter model. It's simple, but effective. Most of them feature a variety of speeds and rhythms. Many people use this vibe not internally, but on the clitoris. We don't all enjoy vibrations inside the vagina.

Mini vibrator

Clitoral orgasm

The "mini," also known as a bullet vibrator, is small and pocket-sized. That makes it ideal for use with a partner during sex or in the shower (only if it's waterproof, obviously). Given the toy's size, most aren't very powerful and don't produce very strong vibrations. More expensive models, like those from the Fun Factory brand, often pack a lot more power.

Vibrator numbness?

Are you not using your vibrating buddy much for fear of a paralyzed clitoris? Luckily that's a fable. That said, a lengthy session with your vibrator can leave your clitoris temporarily numb. The feeling will return after a couple of hours. But you don't need to worry about sustaining damage to your nerve endings from too much vibration or masturbation.

"The best sex I have ever had was with my vibrator."

Eva Longoria

Thrusting vibrator

Vaginal, A-spot, and P-spot orgasm

No one around, but you fancy the feeling of a thrusting pleasure pump? In recent years, thrusting vibrators have gained in popularity. Using a special pulsating technique, the tip moves up and down or back and forth. They are available in smaller sizes with a slight curve for G-spot stimulation. For a mixed orgasm you can use another toy on your clit. If you want to treat yourself, a great option is the Stronic range made by Fun Factory. It's a bit pricey, but it's worth it!

> ## *Quickie*
> **Apply a drop of water-based lubricant to your toy so it slides in better. Please note, however: Silicone lube and silicone sex toys can react with each other.**

Tarzan

Clitoral, vaginal, anal, and/or mixed orgasm

A Tarzan can do it all: It pampers your vagina and clitoris simultaneously and some have an attachment for mild stimulation of your back door. When you don't feel the need for penetration, you can turn the Tarzan over and place the rabbit/dolphin/butterfly on your clitoris.

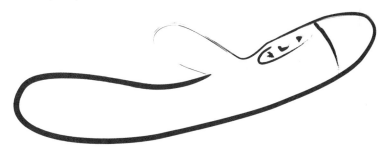

G-spot vibrator

G-spot orgasm

Can't reach your own G-spot or want to apply more pressure? Use a special G-spot vibe. They have a curved tip for maximum hotspot stimulation. To simulate the "come here" motion of your finger you simply move the vibrator up and down.

Clitoris stimulators

Clitoral orgasm

The Rolls Royce among sex toys is the clitoris stimulator. When you place the attachment onto your clitoris it will create a mild vacuum. Instead of vibrations, they rely on pulsating and sucking air pressure waves. The result? Powerful tingling you can feel deep down! Luxury erotica brand LELO even offers an orgasm guarantee on its SONA (which, unlike other styles, uses intense sonic waves). They cost a bomb, but you'll have years of mind-blowing orgasms to look forward to. The Satisfyer stimulators are less mind-blowing, but also pretty good and more affordable.

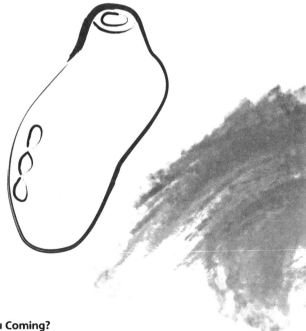

Zumio

Clitoral orgasm

Like the air pressure stimulators, the Zumio yields an entirely different experience compared to most vibrators. The tip of the Zumio toy doesn't vibrate, it oscillates. That is, it moves back and forth incredibly fast. It's so intense that direct stimulation—even at setting 1—is too much for most people. The advice is to place the tip of the Zumio an inch or two away from your clitoris. Even there you'll still feel it!

Quickie
Is even the lowest setting too intense? Place the vibrating toy over your underwear or another piece of fabric.

Nipple clamps

Nipple orgasm

Those with sensitive nipples should give nipple clamps a go. Wear these special "pegs" during sex to put your nerves on edge. You determine the intensity with the help of a small screw. It will bring you another step closer to a nipple orgasm.

Vibrating penis ring

Clitoral orgasm (during penetration)

"A penis ring? What do I need that for?" Because there are vibrating versions. The vibrating part sits on top of the ring and comes into contact with your clitoris during sex. You've guessed it: This increases your chance of coming during penetration. Every time your partner thrusts, you'll feel the vibrations against your clit. Tip: Do the CAT position (page 153). It will maximize contact between the bullet vibe inside the ring and your clitoris. You'll be purring in no time!

Butt plugs

Anal orgasm

Butt plugs for some people might seem tacky, but if you enjoy anal play a plug is a must try. In fact, it feels a bit better, because it doesn't give you the full-on feeling of anal sex. You can use a butt plug as a little extra during sex, including solo. They come in various shapes and sizes: vibrating or not, smooth or ribbed. Beginners are advised to purchase a smooth, short plug. Or else buy a set of different sizes, so you can experiment with the intensity.

Please note: A butt plug should always have a "stopper" at the end. This prevents it from disappearing up your back garden.

Couples toys

Clitoral and vaginal orgasm

Increase your chances of a simultaneous orgasm with a couples toy! These are especially designed for use by couples during sex. Examples include the immensely popular We-Vibe or the LELO Tiani. One end stimulates the glans of the clitoris and the other the G-spot. When your partner also slides in, the toy simply remains in place. With a remote or via an app you can control the intensity and rhythm. Welcome to the future!

You can introduce any kind of vibrator between the sheets. If your partner is a vagina owner, there are also special tools aimed at penetrative sex, but not everyone is into this. The double dildo, for example, enables mutual vaginal stimulation, or you can use a strap-on to penetrate each other. Some versions have a vibrating part for the wearer, so both of you experience pleasure.

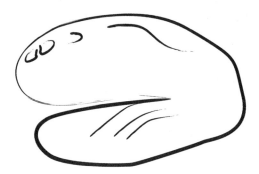

What to look for when buying toys

Beginner? Start small: Don't buy expensive and powerful gadgets when you're a novice in the field of sex toys. You've yet to discover what you like. Start with an entry-level model: a bullet vibrator or a wand vibrator. These are inexpensive. Do you like it? Take it a step further and try a G-spot, Tarzan, or air pressure vibrator.

Buy what suits you: You can buy a handful of random toys to experiment with, but it would be a waste of money if it turns out that half of them are not your thing. Find out what you like in bed. What turns you on the most? Do you enjoy firm and direct stimulation of your clitoris? An air pressure vibrator it is! Do you enjoy double or triple stimulation? Tarzan is your new best friend! Or do you prefer a gentler approach? Opt for a bullet or wand vibrator!

You get what you pay for: This applies to erotic items, too. Cheap toys break more easily, are noisy, not environmentally friendly, often made of material that melts at higher temperatures, and some even contain harmful chemicals. Thirty or forty dollars buys you a good basic toy. At the luxury end, you have to dig deep, but those items are guaranteed to offer years and years of pleasure.

Read reviews: You can't return an intimate product after use. So always read online reviews before you purchase a toy. But bear in mind that what may be unpleasant for one person could be divine for another. At the very least, reviews should be able to tell you whether the manufacturing quality is decent.

Appendix

Orgasm ABCs

Just the basics

Anilingus: licking somebody's anus

Anorgasmia: difficulty or inability reaching orgasm

Big O: popular synonym for orgasm

Coregasm: an orgasm during exercise

Couples toys: sex toys made especially for two people playing together

Cunnilingus: stimulation of the clitoris (and vulva) with the mouth and tongue

Edging: a technique in which you take short breaks to increase the intensity of your eventual orgasm

Erogenous zone: any area on the body that causes arousal when touched in the right way

Foreplay: whatever you want it to be! Sexting, kissing, cuddling, massage, manual sex, oral sex . . .

Glans clitoris: the external part of the clitoris

Happy ending: another word for orgasm

Hysteria: an antiquated, overarching term popular in the Victorian era to describe mental problems among women, including depression, rage, and sexual excess

La petite mort: French expression for orgasm

Manual sex: sexual activity with your hands, including jacking off and fingering

Oral sex: sexual activities with the mouth, including blowing, cunnilingus, and anilingus

Post-sex blues: a sad, somber feeling after sex and/or orgasm

Tantric sex: a form of sex inherited from the Tantra tradition that revolves less around physical aspects and more around connection

Vagina: the internal part of the sexual organ for those assigned female at birth—or, for some people, post–gender confirmation surgery (then, sometimes referred to as a neovagina)

Vaginismus: a condition in which the vagina doesn't allow penetration: no penis, and often not even a tampon

Vulva: the external part of the sexual organ for those assigned female at birth, including the labia, glands, clitoris, and openings of the urethra and vagina

Further Reading and Resources

BOOKS

Come as You Are: The Surprising New Science That Will Transform Your Sex Life by Emily Nagoski, PhD

Tantric Orgasm for Women by Diana Richardson

The Multi-Orgasmic Woman: Discover Your Full Desire, Pleasure, and Vitality by Mantak Chia and Rachel Carlton Adams, MD

The Game of Desire: 5 Surprising Secrets of Dating with Dominance—and Getting What You Want by Shan Boodram

Becoming Cliterate: Why Orgasm Equality Matters—And How to Get It by Laurie Mintz, PhD

The Vagina Bible: The Vulva and the Vagina—Separating the Myth from the Medicine by Jen Gunter, MD

Doing It: Women Tell the Truth About Great Sex by Karen Pickering

What You Really Really Want: The Smart Girl's Shame-Free Guide to Sex and Safety by Jaclyn Friedman

The Cosmo Kama Sutra: 99 Mind-Blowing Sex Positions by the editors of *Cosmopolitan*

Mating in Captivity: Unlocking Erotic Intelligence by Esther Perel

WEBSITES

LotteLust.com
OMGYES.com
BadGirlsBible.com
TalkTabu.com
SluttyGirl Problems.com
SoundsofPleasure.tumblr.com
xconfessions.com

TV SHOWS AND DOCUMENTARIES

Netflix's *Sex, Explained*
Masters of Sex
Sex Education
#Female Pleasure

PODCASTS

How Cum Podcast
Women Watching Porn
Where Should We Begin with Esther Perel
Sex with Emily
I Want It That Way: Bustle on Sex and Relationships
Guys We F****d
Savage Lovecast

Acknowledgments

This book wouldn't have come about without help from the many amazing people who, like us at LotteLust, are keen to break taboos and reduce the orgasm gap: Barbara Carrellas, Lorrae Jo Bradbury, Dorian Solot, and Marla Renee Stewart. They are all keen to break taboos and to reduce the orgasm gap. And it wouldn't have happened without you either, Marjolein Abma, LotteLust's in-house sexologist!

Our thanks also to the strong women who were willing to describe their orgasms, to Bo Sterenberg for her beautiful illustrations, and to Kosmos Uitgevers—in particular, Marieke and Levi—for giving us a chance to write and publish this book.

Last but not least: A big thanks to The Experiment for their incredible skills and enthusiasm—and for taking us and this book on an exciting international journey.

About the Author

Laura Hiddinga is a journalist and writes for LotteLust, an online magazine for womxn who want to learn about sexuality, have fun, and fantasize. She lives in Amsterdam, in the Netherlands—a country widely regarded as boasting the most progressive sex education and sexual values in the world.

LotteLust.com